OXFORD SPECIALTY

BMA

Clinical SAQs for the Final FRCEM

D1354658

OXFORD SPECIALTY TRAINING

Clinical SAQs for the Final FRCEM

Ashis Banerjee
Consultant in Emergency Medicine, Royal Free London NHS Foundation Trust,
Barnet Hospital

Anisa J. N. Jafar
Specialist registrar in emergency medicine
North West Deanery, England

Angshuman Mukherjee
Consultant in Emergency Medicine, Royal Free London NHS Foundation Trust,
Barnet Hospital

Christian Solomonides
Consultant in Emergency Medicine, Royal Free London NHS Foundation Trust,
Barnet Hospital

Erik Witt
Consultant in Emergency Medicine, Royal Free London NHS Foundation Trust,
Barnet Hospital

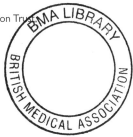

OXFORD
UNIVERSITY PRESS

Great Clarendon Street, Oxford, OX2 6DP,
United Kingdom

Oxford University Press is a department of the University of Oxford.
It furthers the University's objective of excellence in research, scholarship,
and education by publishing worldwide. Oxford is a registered trade mark of
Oxford University Press in the UK and in certain other countries

First Edition published in 2019

Impression: 1

Published in the United States of America by Oxford University Press
198 Madison Avenue, New York, NY 10016, United States of America

British Library Cataloguing in Publication Data
Data available

Library of Congress Control Number: 2019948078

ISBN 978–0–19–881467–2

Printed in Great Britain by
Bell & Bain Ltd., Glasgow

Contents

Abbreviations

ABCDE	Airway, Breathing, Circulation, Disability, Exposure
ACE	angiotensin-converting enzymes
ACEI	angiotensin-converting enzyme inhibitor
ACS	acute coronary syndrome
ALS	advanced life support
ANC	absolute neutrophil count
ASIS	anterior superior iliac spine
ATRIA	Anticoagulation and Risk Factors in Atrial Fibrillation
AV	atrioventricular
BCSH	British Committee for Standards in Haematology
BNF	British National Formulary
CARLS	cyanosis, air entry, retractions, level of consciousness, saturation
CATS	children's acute transport service
CIWA	Clinical Institute Withdrawal Assessment
CNS	central nervous system
COPD	chronic obstructive pulmonary disease
CPAP	continuous positive airway pressure
CPR	cardiopulmonary resuscitation
CRP	C-reactive protein
CRVO	central retinal vein occlusion
CT	computed tomography
DBP	diastolic blood pressure
DVLA	Driver and Vehicle Licensing Agency
ECG	electrocardiogram
ED	emergency department
EM	erythema migrans
ENT	ear, nose, throat
ESC	European Society of Cardiology
FFP	fresh frozen plasma
GABA	gamma-aminobutyric acid
GCS	Glasgow Coma Score
HA	hereditary angioedema
HELLP	haemolysis, elevated liver enzymes, and low platelet count
HEMS	Helicopter Emergency Medical Service
HFA	Heart Failure Association
HHS	hyperosmolar hyperglycaemic state
HSP	Henoch–Schönlein purpura
HZO	herpes zoster ophthalmicus
IBD	inflammatory bowel disease
ICD	implantable cardioverter defibrillator
ICP	intracranial pressure
INR	international normalized ratio
IRAD	International Registry of Acute Aortic Dissection
IVC	inferior vena cava
NICE	National Institute for Health and Care Excellence
NIHSS	NIH Stroke Severity Score

NSAID	non-steroidal anti-inflammatory drug
NSTE-ACS	non-ST-elevation acute coronary syndrome
ORIF	open reduction and internal fixation
PE	pulmonary embolism
PEEP	positive end-expiratory pressure
PEG	percutaneous endoscopic gastrostomy
PERC	Pulmonary Embolism Rule-Out Criteria
PID	pelvic inflammatory disease
PPE	personal protective equipment
PRISM	primary care streptococcal management
qSOFA	quick Sequential Organ Failure Assessment
RCOG	Royal College of Obstetricians and Gynaecologists
ROSIER	Recognition of Stroke in the Emergency Room
RSI	rapid sequence induction
RVO	retinal vein occlusion
SAH	subarachnoid haemorrhage
SAQ	short answer questions
SAU	surgical assessment unit
SBP	systolic blood pressure (also spontaneous bacterial peritonitis)
SJS	Steven–Johnson syndrome
SM	sartorius muscle
SOFA	Sequential Organ Failure Assessment
TBS	total body surface
TEN	toxic epidermal necrolysis
TIA	transient ischaemic attack
VOR	vestibulo-ocular reflex
WHO	World Health Organization

Introduction

The Final FRCEM examination is a high-stakes event, successful completion of which forms part of the requirements for obtaining a Certificate of Completion of Training in the specialty of Emergency Medicine in the United Kingdom. A new examination format was introduced on 1 August 2016.

The purpose of this book is to acquaint emergency medicine trainees with the format and potential content of the Short Answer Question (SAQ) paper in the Final FRCEM examination subsequent to introduction of the above-mentioned changes.

The Final FRCEM SAQ section comprises 60 questions to be answered in a period of three hours with 3 marked questions. In this book each practice SAQ has 3 parts and these are worth 1 mark each—this may differ in the FRCEM exam itself where some SAQs may have parts worth 2 marks. The extent of knowledge required for a successful outcome is wide ranging as is, indeed, the scope of emergency medicine as a specialty. There is no substitute to acquiring a solid grounding in the relevant areas of the curriculum.

While answering the SAQ paper, it is important to have a good time management strategy. Questions that appear difficult should ideally be answered towards the end after completion of the bulk of the paper.

Candidates may find this book useful in the achievement of a successful outcome, alongside self-preparation, guided by standard textbooks, online revision courses, and attendance at SAQ courses. The provided answers are inevitably of greater length than feasible in the real examination to enable provision of additional factual material. The Royal College of Emergency Medicine website provides authoritative guidance regarding the examination and must be consulted as a matter of necessity.

We wish our readers the best as they prepare for this exam.

Acknowledgements

We are grateful to Geraldine Jeffers for suggesting this project, and Rachel Goldsworthy, both of Oxford University Press, for their support and oversight of this project.

Ashis Banerjee
Anisa Jafar
Angshuman Mukherjee
Christian Solomonides
Erik Witt

Chapter 1 **Abdominal Surgery**

SAQ 1 **Abdominal Pain**

An 82-year-old male presents with generalized abdominal pain and distension which has progressed over the preceding four days. Fig. 1.1 shows his abdominal radiograph.

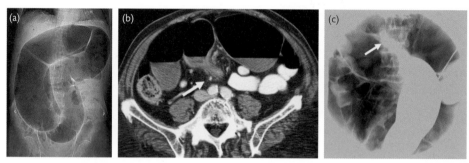

Fig. 1.1 Reproduced from Levy, A., Mortele, K. and Yeh, B. (2015). *Gastrointestinal Imaging*. Oxford University Press USA. Copyright © 2017 Oxford University Press. Reproduced with permission of the Licensor through PLSclear.

Q1. What is the diagnosis? List one possible underlying cause and two complications of this condition.

Q2. How can this be managed acutely?

Q3. List four medical causes of acute abdominal pain.

Answers

A1.

The colon is dilated and does not display haustral markings. The features are those of a closed-loop large bowel obstruction, suggesting sigmoid volvulus, which is the commonest type of volvulus involving the gastrointestinal tract. The dilated sigmoid colon is often described as demonstrating a coffee bean appearance, caused by central notching. Potential underlying causes include chronic constipation and/or laxative abuse, chronic neurological disease (e.g. Parkinson's disease and multiple sclerosis), and psychotropic medication (e.g. for chronic schizophrenia). The redundant and mobile sigmoid colon undergoes torsion, usually in a clockwise direction, around its mesenteric axis. The root of the sigmoid mesocolons is usually narrowed. Complications include (choose two from):

- Strangulation leading to gangrene
- Bowel perforation
- Faecal peritonitis
- Recurrent volvulus

A2.

The patient is placed in the left lateral position and a sigmoidoscope (along with a rectal flatus tube) is fed into the twisted loop to decompress it, allowing detorsion. Without definitive surgery, usually performed electively and involving sigmoid resection, 60% will recur. Emergency surgery is required in the presence of bowel gangrene.

A3.

Medical causes of acute abdominal pain include (choose four from):

- Henoch–Schönlein purpura
  - Necrotizing vasculitis of arterioles and capillaries, most common in male children and with abdominal pain, haematuria/proteinuria, and joint pain as classical manifestations
- Hypercalcaemia
  - Most commonly this is caused by malignancy or primary hyperparathyroidism
- Lower lobe pneumonia
  - This further makes the case for performing chest radiography in adults with undiagnosed upper abdominal pain
- Inferior myocardial infarction
  - Electrocardiogram (ECG) is likely to show ST elevation in leads II, III, and aVF with ST depression in lateral+/– high lateral leads (I, aVL, V5, V6)
- Acute intermittent porphyria
  - Metabolic disorder with dysfunctional production of haem
- Diabetic ketoacidosis
  - The cause of abdominal pain in this circumstance is not definitively known but is likely related to a level of gastroparesis influenced by the metabolic disturbance
- Lead poisoning
  - For symptoms such as abdominal pain to appear, dangerous blood levels are likely to have been reached
- Opiate withdrawal
  - There are multiple different management modalities for this such as antidepressants, benzodiazepines, clonidine, laxatives, and psychological interventions
- Addison's disease
  - This is primary adrenal insufficiency causing low cortisol
- Sickle cell crisis
  - Although pain can be caused by vascular occlusion, a different underlying cause of the pain (such as appendicitis) may be the trigger for the crisis itself

Further Reading

Tiah L, Goh SH. Sigmoid volvulus: diagnostic twists and turns. *European Journal of Emergency Medicine.* 2006;13(2):84–7.
Tidy C (2015). *Sigmoid Volvulus 2015.* Available from: http://patient.info/doctor/sigmoid-volvulus

SAQ 2 **Post-laparoscopy Complications**

A 23-year-old female presents with severe abdominal pain following diagnostic laparoscopy, at which endometriosis has been diagnosed.

Q1. List at least six features which might suggest a postoperative complication of laparoscopic surgery.

Q2. After some time in the department, you become concerned that this lady might be suffering a complication. Which two diagnostic approaches are appropriate to assess this?

Q3. What is meant by abdominal compartment syndrome?

Answers

A1.

Features suggesting a complication of laparoscopic surgery include:

- abdominal pain needing opiate analgesia
- anorexia or reluctance to drink
- reluctance to mobilize
- nausea
- vomiting
- tachycardia
- abdominal tenderness
- abdominal distension
- poor urine output
- cardiac arrhythmia

The National Patient Safety Association produced a report discussing missed complications of laparoscopic surgery and cited these ten indicators as something which should raise suspicion and possibly prompt senior surgical review.

A2.

Computed tomography (CT) scan and/or diagnostic laparoscopy are indicated to assess the cause of the presentation. Ultrasound is unlikely to be useful in the presence of free gas in the abdomen as it will prevent a good image.

A3.

Abdominal compartment syndrome refers to increased pressure within the abdomen usually due to oedema, accumulation of free fluid, or distension of the bowel, such that the compliance threshold of the abdomen is breached and the abdominal wall can no longer stretch. This is associated with organ dysfunction related to the consequent intra-abdominal hypertension. Organ dysfunction occurs in the presence of a sustained intra-abdominal pressure greater than 20 mm Hg. Normally, intra-abdominal pressure ranges between 5 and 7 mm Hg, and intra-abdominal hypertension is diagnosed with a pressure greater than 12 mm Hg.

Further Reading

Kapadia CR, McMahon MJ. Guidelines on the management of complications. Association of Laparoscopic Surgeons of Great Britain and Ireland. Clinical Guidelines, ALSGBI, 2006

NPSA. Laparoscopic surgery: failure to recognise post-operative deterioration. London, UK: National Patient Safety Agency. 2010.

SAQ 3 **Cholangitis**

A 38-year-old man presents with right upper quadrant abdominal pain and confusion. He is pyrexial. You make a preliminary diagnosis of acute ascending cholangitis.

Q1. Name two organisms that may be involved.
Q2. List three predisposing factors for the development of this condition.
Q3. What triad of diagnostic features typically is associated with cholangitis?

Answers

A1.

Potential causative organisms include:

- *Escherichia coli*
- Klebsiella
- Enterococci
- Pseudomonas aeruginosa
- *Enterobacter*
- Streptococci

A2.

Predisposing factors for cholangitis include:

- Gallstones
- Intestinal parasites
- Biliary tree instrumentation: ERCP
- Biliary stricture
- Neoplasm (ampulla of Vater, common bile duct, duodenum, head of pancreas, gallbladder)
- AIDS

A3.

The triad indicating cholangitis comprises:

- Right upper quadrant pain
- Jaundice
- Fever, usually with chills or rigors

At least half to over a third of presentations involve this triad and up to another fifth presents with the Reynolds pentad, which adds shock and an altered mental state to this classic Charcot's triad.

Ideally blood cultures ought to be taken before antibiotics are administered with Gram-negative and anaerobic cover. Sometimes endoscopic drainage is required, especially when further organ involvement develops, or the patient develops refractory circulatory shock. Liver abscesses, sepsis, and multiorgan dysfunction can develop as a complication of cholangitis itself. Following any biliary drainage bleeding, fistulae and bile leakage are potential complications.

Further Reading

Miura F, Takada T, Strasberg SM, Solomkin JS, Pitt HA, Gouma DJ, et al. (2013) TG13 flowchart for the management of acute cholangitis and cholecystitis. *Journal of Hepatobiliary and Pancreatic Science.* 2013;20(1):47–54.

SAQ 4 **Acute Appendicitis**

A 17-year-old male presents with acute abdominal pain. You are concerned that he may have acute appendicitis.

Q1. What is the mechanism by which appendicitis is believed to occur and what risk factors exist for its development?

Q2. Describe two atypical anatomical presentations of appendicitis.

Q3. Name a scoring system which may be useful in arriving at the diagnosis and the salient features of this scoring system.

Answers

A1.

It is thought that appendicitis represents secondary infection following obstruction of the appendiceal lumen. Potential causes which may lead to luminal obstruction can be:

- Faecoliths
- Submucosal lymphoid hyperplasia as a result of viral infection
- Undigestible food fragments
- Parasites
- Tumour growth, such as adenocarcinoma of the caecum, or carcinoid

Risk factors for developing appendicitis include:

- Age—there is a peak in incidence between the age of 10 and 20 years; however, any age group can develop appendicitis.
- Men—more males than females develop appendicitis by a ratio of 1.4:1.
- Antibiotic use—frequent antibiotics can alter the flora of the gut to the extent whereby response to viral infections is modified, which then may trigger appendicitis.
- Smoking—this risk is increased in smokers and in children who are passive smokers.

A2.

Atypical presentations of appendicitis can be seen in the following situations related to altered anatomical position:

- Pregnancy causes a shift in normal anatomy, especially in the latter trimesters—pain may be felt in the right upper quadrant or right flank.
- Retrocaecal appendicitis may result in right loin pain and a positive psoas test (this involves passively extending the right thigh while in the left lateral position, which elicits pain in the right lower quadrant). Overlying caecum can protect from tenderness on deep palpation.
- Pre/post-ileal appendicitis may present as diarrhoea and vomiting.

- Subcaecal/pelvic appendicitis may present with pain in the suprapubic area with urinary frequency. Tenesmus and diarrhoea are possible due to rectal irritation and vaginal tenderness is also possible on the right side. Haematuria and leucocyturia may be noted on urine dipstick testing.
- A long appendix with inflammation at the tip may cause left lower quadrant pain.

A3.

The Alvarado score comprises three symptoms, three signs, and two laboratory findings, with a maximum total score of 10:

- Abdominal pain that migrates to the right lower quadrant (+1)
- Anorexia (+1)
- Nausea or vomiting (+1)
- Right lower quadrant tenderness (+2)
- Nausea or vomiting (+1)
- Rebound tenderness (+1)
- Elevated temperature (>37.3°C) (+1)
- Leukocytosis >10 000 /µL (+2)
- Neutrophilia with left shift (+1)

Reprinted from *Annals of Emergency Medicine*, 15, 5, Alvarado, A. A practical score for the early diagnosis of acute appendicitis. pp. 557–564. https://doi.org/10.1016/S0196-0644(86)80993-3. Copyright © 1986 Published by Mosby, Inc., with permission from Elsevier.
　　There is a very low risk of appendicitis with a score of less than 4 points.

Further Reading

Alvarado A. A practical score for the early diagnosis of acute appendicitis. *Annals of Emergency Medicine*.1986;15(5):557–64.
NICE (2016). *Appendicitis—CKS 2016*. Available from: https://cks.nice.org.uk/appendicitis#!topicsummary

SAQ 5 **Acute Cholecystitis**

A 32-year-old female presents to you with right upper quadrant pain. She is known to have gallstones and you suspect that this is cholecystitis.

Q1. Give four risk factors for gallstone formation
Q2. What are the clinical features you look for when diagnosing cholecystitis? Give at least four
Q3. Give two possible complications of acute cholecystitis

Answers

A1.

Risk factors for gallstone formation include any four from:

- Female sex
- Older age
- Obesity
- Rapid weight loss over a short period
- Pregnancy
- Crohn's disease
- Hyperlipidaemia
- Diabetes mellitus (metabolic syndrome of type 2 diabetes mellitus, truncal obesity, insulin resistance, hypertension, and hyperlipidaemia)
- Family history of gall stones
- Haemolytic disorders (pigment gallstones)

A2.

Signs and symptoms of acute cholecystitis include (give four from):

- Sudden onset right upper quadrant pain which is constant and severe
- Anorexia
- Nausea and vomiting
- Fever (usually low grade)
- Tender right upper quadrant with a positive Murphy's sign, which has a specificity of over 79% (this is pain on palpation of the right upper quadrant which inhibits inspiration)
- Gallstones in the history

Raised white cell count and C-reactive protein are commonly found. Other differential diagnoses to be aware of include peptic ulcer disease, hepatitis, pancreatitis, and cardiac disease. It is important to try to rule them out with history, physical examination, and investigations as appropriate.

A3.

Complications of acute cholecystitis include (give two from):

- Gallbladder perforation
- Biliary peritonitis
- Development of pericholecystic abscess
- Development of fistula between the gallbladder and duodenum

Although mortality is less than 10%, in older people it is higher and comorbidities (such as diabetes mellitus) worsen prognosis.

Further Reading

Elwood DR. Cholecystitis. *Surgical Clinics of North America*. 2008;88(6):1241–52, viii.
NICE. *Cholecystitis—Acute—CKS*. 2013. Available from: https://cks.nice.org.uk/cholecystitis-acute

SAQ 6 Ingested Foreign Body

Worried parents bring their three-year-old son into the emergency department, concerned that their child may have a coin stuck in the throat. See Fig. 1.2.

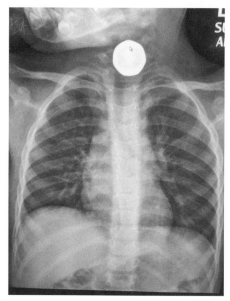

Fig. 1.2

Q1. Please consider the choking algorithm. If this conscious child has an ineffective cough, what are the next steps?
Q2. With gastrointestinal foreign bodies, where are the high-risk areas for impaction?
Q3. List three possible complications of foreign body ingestion.

Answers

A1.

The recommended sequence of actions includes:

1. Five back blows initially
2. Five thrusts (chest for infant, abdominal for child >1 year)
3. If the child is unconscious, the next step would be to open the airway, give five rescue breaths, and commence cardiopulmonary resuscitation

A2.

Foreign body impaction in the gastrointestinal tract occurs preferentially at either:

- Upper oesophageal sphincter
- Lower oesophageal sphincter
- Pylorus

This coin is likely to be in the oesophagus, as it projects *en face*, appearing round, in the anteroposterior view. A coin in the trachea appears in the sagittal plane (end on) in this projection.

Radiography is only useful for radio-opaque items (unless there are concerns about perforation, for example). It should be remembered that bottle caps and can rings do not always show up, however, they are potentially problematic if not investigated. Endoscopy is important in cases where sharp, large, long, oddly shaped (likely to obstruct) objects have been swallowed.

A3.

Complications of foreign body ingestion include (choose three from):

- Laceration of mucosal surfaces
- Stricture
- Perforation (subsequent mediastinitis/pneumothorax/pericarditis/cardiac tamponade/peritonitis)
- Abscess formation
- Fistula formation
- Bowel necrosis
- Heavy metal poisoning

It is well known that button batteries are especially concerning because of their increased size resulting in much more likely oesophageal impaction, and the increasing use of lithium means that a higher voltage is carried. A release of hydroxide radicals at the site causes a caustic mucosal injury due to an increase in pH.

One key element of the consultation must be to document and address any home circumstances which may have led to the child being able to ingest a foreign body. Clearly young children are prone to such events; however, it must at least be in the clinician's mind to seek for evidence of neglect/chaotic living. Furthermore, especially in an older child, deliberate ingestion must be investigated appropriately.

Further Reading

Kramer RE, Lerner DG, Lin T, Manfredi M, Shah M, Stephen TC, et al. Management of ingested foreign bodies in children: a clinical report of the NASPGHAN Endoscopy Committee. *Journal of Pediatric Gastroenterology and Nutrition*. 2015;60(4):562–74.

Resuscitation Council UK. *Paediatric Choking Algorithm*. 2015. Available from: https://www.resus.org.uk/resuscitation-guidelines/paediatric-basic-life-support/#choking

SAQ 7 **Abdominal Pain and Vomiting**

A patient presents with abdominal pain and vomiting. Her abdominal radiograph is shown in Fig. 1.3.

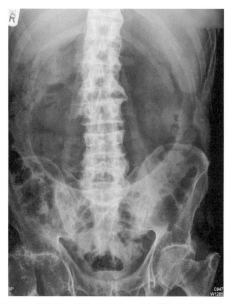

Fig. 1.3 Reproduced from Thomas, W., Reed, M. and Wyatt, M. (2016). *Oxford Textbook of Fundamentals of Surgery*. Oxford: Oxford University Press. © Oxford University Press 2016. Reproduced with permission of the Licensor through PLSclear.

Q1. What does the radiograph show?

Q2. What causes this presentation?

Q3. What is the management?

Answers

A1.

The X-ray shows gastric volvulus.

Some features to look out for on a radiograph include:

- A stomach which appears to be 'upside down'
- A fluid level behind the cardiac shadow
- A double air-fluid level
- An overly large and distended stomach
- Collapse of the small bowel distal to the volvulus

A2.

Gastric volvulus can be:

Primary: related to neoplasia, adhesions, or abnormal attachments of stomach (due to ligament anomalies);

Secondary to disorders of gastric anatomy/gastric function; abnormalities of adjacent organs (diaphragm, spleen); or occurring in association, in adults, with a para-oesophageal hernia/ traumatic defects/diaphragmatic eventration/ phrenic nerve paralysis.

A3.

Initial treatment includes keeping the patient prone and inserting a nasogastric tube to facilitate compression. Surgical involvement is needed immediately if the diagnosis is acute, because of the risk of vascular compromise and mortality. Surgical and/or conservative approaches have been used successfully. The most frequently reported surgery is open surgical reduction +/– gastropexy, although laparoscopic approaches/endoscopic reduction as well as a percutaneous endoscopic gastrostomy (PEG) tube can be used. In older people or those with chronic gastric volvulus, conservative approaches are more commonly adopted.

Further Reading

Rashid F, Thangarajah T, Mulvey D, Larvin M, Iftikhar SY. A review article on gastric volvulus: a challenge to diagnosis and management. *International Journal of Surgery*. 2010;8(1):18–24.

Tillman BW, Merritt NH, Emmerton-Coughlin H, Mehrotra S, Zwiep T, Lim R (2014). Acute gastric volvulus in a six-year-old: a case report and review of the literature. *Journal of Emergency Medicine*. 2014;46(2):191–6.

SAQ 8 **Rectal Bleeding**

A 24-year-old female presents with severe pain and rectal bleeding.

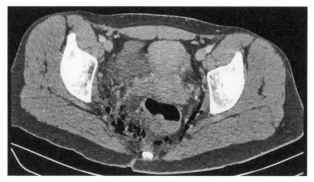

Fig. 1.4

Q1. What is the abnormality seen in the CT scan (Fig. 1.4)?

Q2. What is the likely diagnosis?

Q3. List three management priorities.

Answers

A1.

The CT scan shows extensive retroperitoneal gas within the presacral space and tissues surrounding the rectum.

A2.

The likely diagnosis is rectal perforation.

A3.

Management comprises the following:

• Fluid resuscitation
• Intravenous analgesia
• Intravenous broad-spectrum antibiotics
• Nil by mouth
• Urgent surgical referral

Rectal perforation can be iatrogenic (related to instrumentation or enema administration), or associated with rectal prolapse, diverticular disease, neoplasm, blunt or penetrating trauma (including auto-erotic activity), ulcerative colitis, or stercoral ulceration.

Rectal bleeding is usually caused by benign conditions (e.g. anal fissures, haemorrhoids especially in those under 30 years of age). However, there are other possible causes, such as inflammatory bowel disease (again, more likely in the under 30s), neoplastic disease (more suspicious in the over 50s), diverticulitis, polyps, radiation proctitis, gastroenteritis, angiodysplasia, ischaemic colitis, rectal ulceration, sexually transmitted infections, and anorectal trauma.

The first-line treatment for anal fissures is glyceryl trinitrate ointment followed by topical diltiazem at 2%. Other options include botulinum toxin injection, fistulectomy, and sphincterotomy.

Radiation proctitis does not respond well to many topical treatments except rectal sucralfate enemas. Argon plasma coagulation is the ultimate management for this.

Further Reading

Banerjee A, Oliver C. Surgery. In: *Revision Notes for the FRCEM Intermediate SAQ Paper*, Chapter 6. Oxford, UK: Oxford University Press; 2017.
Royal College of Surgeons. *Commissioning Guide: Rectal Bleeding*. London, UK: Royal College of Surgeons; 2013

Chapter 2 **Cardiology**

SAQ 1 **Acute Coronary Syndrome**

A 73-year-old female is diagnosed with Takotsubo cardiomyopathy, following presentation with chest pain and ST elevation on a 12-lead electrocardiogram (ECG)

Q1. List three of the most frequent causes of raised troponin other than acute myocardial infarction or Takotsubo cardiomyopathy.

Q2. If this patient did not have ST elevation and was awaiting troponin results, she would clinically fit the NSTE-ACS (non-ST-elevation acute coronary syndrome) category. In that scenario, what should her ACS drug treatment have been pending the troponin result?

Q3. List at least two high-risk criteria which, according to optimal management guidance, would mandate invasive management (i.e. angiography with or without revascularization) of NSTE-ACS in less than two hours from first clinical contact.

Answers

A1.

Choose three other causes of raised troponin from:

- Tachyarrhythmia
- Heart failure
- Hypertensive emergencies
- Critical illness (such as shock/sepsis/burns)
- Myocarditis
- Structural heart disease (such as aortic stenosis)
- Aortic dissection
- Pulmonary embolism
- Pulmonary hypertension
- Renal dysfunction alongside cardiac disease

Takotsubo cardiomyopathy is also referred to as 'apical ballooning' and is widely considered to be a cardiomyopathy triggered by extreme emotional stress. The features include chest pain, raised troponin, often a normal angiogram, and some left ventricular dysfunction on echocardiography (appearing similar to acute myocardial infarction), which is both acute and transient. Angiography must be performed regardless of diagnostic suspicion to rule out a coronary aetiology. Around 75% of those with Takotsubo cardiomyopathy have a high catecholamine level and therefore some dysfunction of the vasculature, which then leads to microvascular spasm and is purported as the mechanism of the disease. Formal diagnosis and treatment of the condition remains without consensus.

A2.

Aspirin and parenteral anticoagulant (usually a low-molecular weight heparin or fondaparinux) for anticoagulation. If NSTE-ACS was then established and the patient was not intended for urgent intervention and did not represent a high bleeding risk, ticagrelor should be added.

A3.

Two high-risk criteria would include:

- Haemodynamic instability/cardiogenic shock
- Recurrent/ongoing chest pain refractory to medical management
- Life-threatening arrhythmia/cardiac arrest
- Mechanical complications of myocardial infarction
- Acute cardiac failure
- Recurrent dynamic ST-T wave change

The European Society of Cardiology has up-to-date guidance on the optimal timing of invasive management of patients with NSTE-ACS depending on presence/absence of specific risk-level features.

Further Reading

Roffi M, Patrono C, Collet JP, Mueller C, Valgimigli M, Andreotti F, et al. 2015 ESC Guidelines for the management of acute coronary syndromes in patients presenting without persistent ST-segment elevation: Task Force for the Management of Acute Coronary Syndromes in Patients Presenting without Persistent ST-Segment Elevation of the European Society of Cardiology (ESC). *European Heart Journal*. 2016;37(3):267–315.

Sharkey SW, Lesser JR, Maron BJ (2011). Cardiology patient page. Takotsubo (stress) cardiomyopathy. *Circulation*. 2011;124(18):e460–2.

SAQ 2 **CHA2-DS2-VASc Score**

A 65-year-old woman presents in atrial fibrillation. She has been feeling 'not quite right' for a week or so, with fluttering feelings in her chest. She has a past medical history of hypertension, but does not seem to have a precipitating cause for atrial fibrillation.

Q1. Based on the CHA2-DS2-VASc Score, would you be recommending that this lady is anticoagulated?

Q2. Why might the CHADS2 score be less preferable for use in an emergency department?

Q3. What is the Anticoagulation and Risk Factors in Atrial Fibrillation (ATRIA) score?

Answers

A1.

Yes. She scores 3 on the calculator, and therefore without other contraindications, anticoagulation should be offered. She has just under 5% risk per year of stroke/TIA/systemic embolism.

The score is made up as follows:

- Age: <65 = 0 Age: 65–74 = 1 Age: 75+ = 2
- Male = 0 Female = 1
- Congestive heart failure = 1
- Hypertension = 1
- History of stroke/TIA/thromboembolism = 2
- History of vascular disease = 1
- Diabetes mellitus = 1

Reprinted from Chest, 137, 2, Lip G.Y. et al. Refining clinical risk stratification for predicting stroke and thromboembolism in atrial fibrillation using a novel risk factor-based approach: the euro heart survey on atrial fibrillation. pp. 263-72. https://doi.org/10.1378/chest.09-1584. Copyright © 2010 The American College of Chest Physicians. Published by Elsevier Inc. All rights reserved. With permission from Elsevier.

A2.

The CHADS2 score misses some higher risk patients, therefore a score of 0 could still mean a yearly risk of 3.2% for stroke if a patient is left without anticoagulation.

A3.

The ATRIA score is a tool used to predict warfarin-associated haemorrhage, and looks at several parameters, outlined in Table 2.1.

Table 2.1

Risk factor	Point value
Anaemia	+3
Severe renal disease/dialysis	+3
Age ≥ 75	+2
Stroke history	+1
Prior haemorrhage	+1
Hypertension	+1

Low risk is considered to be a score less than 4.

In comparison, the HAS-BLED score was considered to perform better and looks at several parameters outlined in Table 2.2.

Table 2.2

Risk factor	Point value
Hypertension	1
Abnormal liver function	1
Abnormal renal function	1
Stroke history	1
Bleeding predisposition	1
Labile INRs	1
Elderly (age >65)	1
Drug/alcohol usage	1

Here a score or 3 or more should prompt a clinician to consider alternatives to anticoagulation as bleeding risk is high. A score of 2 represents moderate risk and therefore close monitoring of further risk factors will need to be taken if the patient is to be anticoagulated.

Further Reading

Lip GY, Nieuwlaat R, Pisters R, Lane DA, Crijns HJ. Refining clinical risk stratification for predicting stroke and thromboembolism in atrial fibrillation using a novel risk factor-based approach: the Euro Heart Survey on atrial fibrillation. Chest. 2010;137(2):263–72.

MDCalc. *CHA$_2$DS$_2$-VASc Score for Atrial Fibrillation Stroke Risk.* 2016. Available from: http://www.mdcalc.com/cha2ds2-vasc-score-atrial-fibrillation-stroke-risk/

MDCalc. *HAS-BLED Score for Major Bleeding Risk.* 2016. Available from: http://www.mdcalc.com/has-bled-score-major-bleeding-risk/#about-equation

SAQ 3 **Echo Image**

Q1. What is the diagnosis in Fig. 2.1?

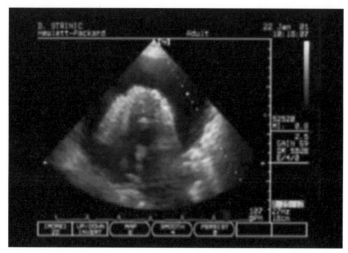

Fig. 2.1 Reproduced from Lancellotti, P., Zamorano, J., Habib, G. and Badano, L. (2016). *The EACVI Textbook of Echocardiography*. 2nd ed. Oxford University Press. © European Society of Cardiology 2017. Reproduced with permission of the Licensor through PLSclear.

Q2. What are the possible causes?

Q3. What is the most urgent concern in this patient and how do you detect it?

Answers

A1.

The diagnosis is pericardial effusion, as demonstrated by a circumferential echo-free space surrounding the heart, and between the parietal and visceral layers of the pericardium. Epicardial fat presents as a hypoechoic space anterior to the right ventricle.

A2.

There are many potential causes of pericardial effusion:

- Infectious
  - Viral (Coxsackie virus; echovirus; adenovirus; cytomegalovirus; Epstein–Barr virus; mumps; rubella; parvovirus B19; HIV, and so on)
  - Bacterial (staphylococcus; streptococcus; Neisseria usually)
  - Mycobacterial: tuberculosis
  - Fungal
  - Parasitic

- Immune-mediated (systemic lupus erythematosus; Dressler's syndrome; drug-induced; amyloid; granulomatosis with polyangiitis)
- Endocrine (hypothyroidism)
- Neoplastic (metastatic malignancy)
- Cardiac (aortic dissection/heart failure/post-cardiac surgery or intervention)
- Traumatic
- Renal (uraemia)

Acute or subacute pericardial effusions are considered to be those present for less than 3 months, with chronic effusions present for longer. There is a variable approach to classifying an effusion as large or small, however if the total of anterior and posterior echo-absent space comes to more than 20 mm, it is considered to be large.

Depending on the cause, the fluid itself may be serous, purulent, haemorrhagic, chylous, or serosanguinous. This does not help very much in identifying a cause. Instead the categorization of the fluid as transudative or exudative helps narrow the cause down.

Exudates (with high levels of protein (i.e. greater than 3 g/dL), caused by inflammatory processes) include idiopathic, iatrogenic, infectious, malignant, traumatic, cardiorespiratory, and autoimmune processes. A small transudative effusion is not considered to be clinically important.

A3.

The most significant complication is cardiac tamponade, which occurs when a pericardial effusion raises intrapericardial pressure to impair cardiac filling due to chamber compression. This can cause hypotension and cardiovascular collapse. The clinical criteria are:

- Hypotension
- Pulsus paradoxus (fall in systolic blood pressure of 10 mm Hg or more during inspiration)
- Increased jugular venous pressure
- Muffled heart sounds
- Tamponade can be recognized on echocardiography by right atrial systolic collapse, right ventricular diastolic collapse, increased diameter of the inferior vena cava (IVC) with reduced or absent IVC inspiratory inflow leading to loss of respiratory variation

Further Reading

BMJ. *Assessment of Pericardial Effusion*. 2016. Available from: http://bestpractice.bmj.com/best-practice/monograph/458.html

SAQ 4 **Young Chest Pain**

A 19-year-old footballer is brought in by ambulance with sudden onset pleuritic central chest pain while playing. There is no past medical history of note, his observations are normal, and the rhythm strip provided by the ambulance service is seen in Fig. 2.2:

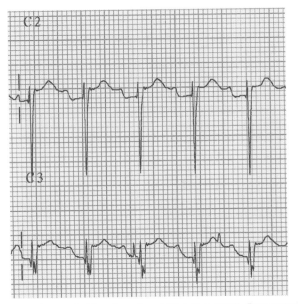

Fig. 2.2 Reproduced from Myerson, S., Choudhury, R. and Mitchell, A. (2010). *Emergencies in Cardiology*. 2nd ed. Oxford: Oxford University Press. © Oxford University Press 2009. Reproduced with permission of the Licensor through PLSclear.

Q1. Describe the rhythm strip in Fig. 2.2 and give the likely diagnosis.
Q2. What beside test would help you evaluate this case and how would you manage the diagnosis?
Q3. List two possible complications.

Answers

A1.

The strip shows sinus rhythm, with PR depression and ST elevation. ST elevation is diffuse, with a concave or saddle-shaped contour. PR depression is very specific for pericarditis (which is the most likely diagnosis in this presentation). PR depression may also be found in atrial ischaemia. In diagnosing acute pericarditis, the patient needs to exhibit two from: chest pain (usually sharp and pleuritic and relieved by sitting forward); a pericardial friction rub on auscultation; complimentary ECG changes (described earlier); a new or worsened pericardial effusion. To move on to a diagnosis of recurrent pericarditis requires a definitive first episode of acute pericarditis (according to the aforementioned criteria), a period of at least 4–6 weeks without any symptoms, good evidence of a recurring picture which involves recurrent pain plus one or more of: pericardial rub on auscultation; complementary ECG changes (described earlier); changes on echocardiography; a new or worsened pericardial effusion; raised white cell count/ESR/CRP (at any level above the laboratory normal range—see further reading).

A2.

Bedside echocardiography (parasternal, four-chamber, or subxiphoid views) would help identify the presence or absence of pericardial effusion. You could recommend non-steroidal anti-inflammatory drugs and colchicine, which reduces the recurrence risk. It is important that the patient is encouraged not to exercise while symptomatic, and competitive athletes should not compete until biomarkers and symptoms have normalized.

A3.

Complications of pericarditis include two from:

- Pericardial effusion
- Cardiac tamponade
- Myopericarditis (which leads to an elevated troponin)
- Chronic constrictive pericarditis

Further Reading

Imazio M, Gaita F, LeWinter M. Evaluation and treatment of pericarditis: a systematic review. *Journal of the American Medical Association*. 2015;314(14):1498–506.

SAQ 5 **Abnormal ECG**

A 48-year-old gentleman attends after three days of diarrhoea and vomiting. He is drowsy and has been moved to the resuscitation room. His ECG is as shown in Fig. 2.3.

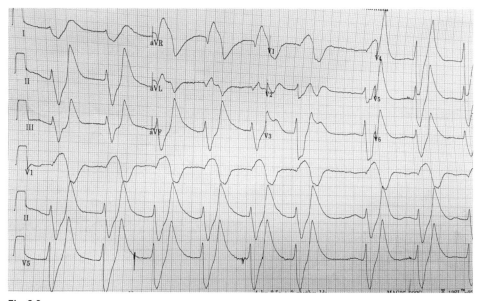

Fig. 2.3

Q1. What does this ECG in Fig. 2.3 show?

Q2. What is the likely underlying cause for this ECG?

Q3. How will you treat this condition in the emergency department?

Answers

A1.

This ECG shows late signs of hyperkalaemia. A broadened QRS complex, flat P, and tall T waves are present. But more importantly the morphology starts to look like a sine wave (hence the name sine wave, which is a preterminal finding).

A2.

The underlying cause for the ECG changes is hyperkalaemia. The first changes of hyperkalaemia are tall T waves and a shortened QT interval. This is followed by progressive lengthening of the PR interval, then of the QRS duration. Eventually the sine wave pattern as just described develops as a preterminal finding.

Causes of hyperkalaemia can be split into those causing impaired renal excretion of potassium such as:

- Acquired hyporeninaemic hypoaldosteronism
- Addison's disease
- Congenital adrenal hyperplasia
- Mineralocorticoid deficiency
- Primary hypoaldosteronism or hyporeninaemia
- Pseudo-hypoaldosteronism
- Renal insufficiency or failure
- Systemic lupus erythematosus
- Type IV renal tubular acidosis
- Most medication causes of hyperkalaemia have an effect on renal excretion

Other causes which result in movement of potassium into the extracellular space include:

- Acidosis
- Damage to tissue from rhabdomyolysis, burns, or trauma
- Familial hyperkalaemic periodic paralysis
- Hyperosmolar states (e.g. uncontrolled diabetes mellitus, glucose infusions)
- Insulin deficiency or resistance
- Tumour lysis syndrome
- Some agents can cause hyperkalaemia by this extracellular mechanism such as: amino acids and packed red blood cells

A3.

A dose of 20 ml 10% calcium gluconate or 10 ml 10% calcium chloride can be used to stabilize the myocardium, while 50 ml of 50% glucose (25 g glucose) with 10 units of short-acting insulin (Actrapid) can help shift the potassium into the cells. Nebulized salbutamol further helps this shift. The current evidence only supports the use of sodium bicarbonate in patients on renal dialysis with severe acidosis.

Further Reading

Hollander-Rodriguez JC, Calvert JF. Hyperkalemia. *American Family Physician*. 2006;73(2):283–90.

SAQ 6 **Bradycardia**

A 72-year-old woman is brought into the resuscitation room with a history of acute onset dizziness. Her blood pressure can only be measured as a systolic of 65 mm Hg, and she appears confused and distressed. The nursing staff have managed to site a cannula.

Q1. What is the diagnosis on the ECG in Fig. 2.4 and what medications could precipitate it?

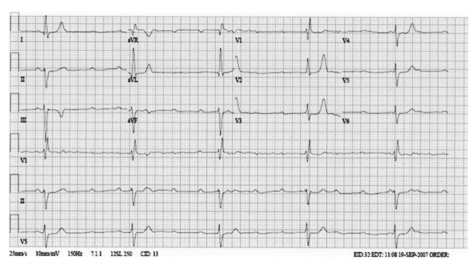

Fig. 2.4 Reproduced from Gray, R. and Pack, L. (2011). *Cardiovascular Disease in the Elderly*. Oxford: Oxford University Press. © Oxford University Press, 2011. Reproduced with permission of the Licensor through PLSclear.

Q2. After your initial ABCDE (Airway, Breathing, Circulation, Disability, Exposure) assessment, placement of monitoring, and full set of observations what is your first-line management?

Q3. Your first-line management is not successful. What are your options now?

Answers

A1.

Complete heart block. This could be precipitated by medications such as: beta-blockers, calcium channel blockers, digoxin. The ECG would concern you more if there was a broad complex and/or ventricular pauses longer than 3 seconds as this would increase the chance of asystole.

A2.

This lady is haemodynamically unstable. First-line measures would be a dose of intravenous atropine 500 mcg. This may then be repeated up to six times (to a maximum of 3 mg). Alternatively, glycopyrronium bromide can be used.

A3.

As the atropine has not been successful, the next step could either be transcutaneous pacing (for which she will require sedation) or intravenous isoprenaline at 5 mcg/minute or intravenous adrenaline 2–10 mcg/min. Other alternatives include aminophylline, dopamine, or glucagon (for beta-adrenergic blocker or calcium channel blocker overdose causing bradycardia).

Further Reading

Resuscitation Council UK. *Adult Bradycardia Algorithm*. 2015. Available from: https://www.resus.org.uk/resuscitation-guidelines/peri-arrest-arrhythmias/#bradycardia

SAQ 7 **Central Crushing Chest Pain**

A 59-year-old gentleman presents with a history of central crushing chest pain. He is now pain free.

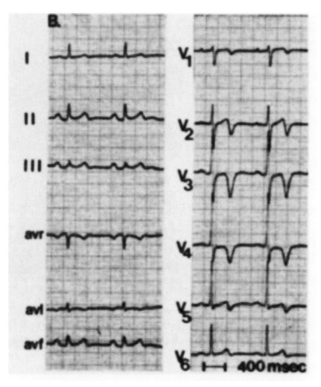

Fig. 2.5 Reprinted from *American Heart Journal*. de Zwaan C, Bär FW, Wellens HJ. Characteristic electrocardiographic pattern indicating a critical stenosis high in left anterior descending coronary artery in patients admitted because of impending myocardial infarction. 1982;103(4 Pt 2):730-6. https://doi.org/10.1016/0002-8703(82)90480-X. Copyright © 1982 Published by Mosby, Inc. With permission from Elsevier.

Q1. Describe the ECG in Fig. 2.5.
Q2. What is the diagnosis?
Q3. What is the likely site of the underlying lesion?

Answers

A1.

The ECG shows deeply inverted T waves in V2–V4.

A2.

The diagnosis is Wellens' syndrome, which is characterized by symmetrical and deep T-wave inversion or biphasic T waves in the anterior precordial leads (leads V2–V4).

A3.

The site of the lesion is likely to be in the left anterior descending coronary artery, where there is severe stenosis. This ECG finding is critical because, despite being pain free at the time and possibly even having normal cardiac markers, the patient is at high risk of extensive anterior myocardial infarction in the coming days/weeks. Furthermore, stress testing can precipitate infarction or cardiac arrest due to the extent of the stenosis, and therefore definitive intervention is required.

Further Reading

de Zwaan C, Bär FW, Wellens HJ. Characteristic electrocardiographic pattern indicating a critical stenosis high in left anterior descending coronary artery in patients admitted because of impending myocardial infarction. *American Heart Journal*. 1982;103(4 Pt 2):730–6.

SAQ 8 **Medical Device**

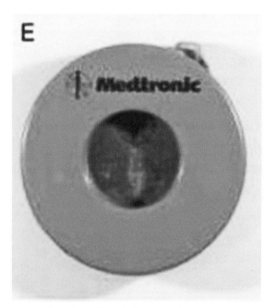

Fig. 2.6 Adapted with permission from Jacob, S. et al. Clinical applications of magnets on cardiac rhythm management devices. *EP Europace*, 13(9), 1222–30. https://doi.org/10.1093/europace/eur137. Copyright © 2011, Oxford University Press.

Q1. What is the device shown in Fig. 2.6?
Q2. What is the indication for its use?
Q3. How is it used?

Answers

A1.

The device is a Medtronic Magnet.

A2.

When a patient with an implantable cardioverter defibrillator (ICD) is at imminent risk of death from misfiring of their ICD, causing multiple shocks to be delivered which were not preceded by ventricular tachycardia or fibrillation. The magnet suspends the detection of tachyarrhythmia, causing no further delivery of shocks.

A3.

Place the magnet on the patient skin over the bump of the ICD (usually left side of chest below the clavicle) and tape in place. The magnet is only effective when in position. Once removed, the ICD reverts to function as before. It is important to leave the magnet in place if a patient dies.

Further Reading

Jacob S, Panaich SS, Maheshwari R, Haddad JW, Padanilam BJ, John SK. Clinical applications of magnets on cardiac rhythm management devices. *Europace*. 2011; 3(9):1222–30.

SAQ 9 **Elderly Chest Pain**

A 75-year-old gentleman attends with shortness of breath, central crushing chest pain, and sweating. His initial observations are heart rate 100/minute, respiratory rate 23/minute, blood pressure 89/54 mm Hg, saturations 95% on a flow rate of 15 litres of oxygen. The ECG shows ST elevation myocardial infarction.

Q1. What is the clinical diagnosis?

Q2. While organizing transfer to a tertiary centre, what treatment would you give to improve the blood pressure?

Q3. If the first treatment is not effective, what pharmacological support could you initiate?

Answers

A1.

The clinical diagnosis is ST elevation myocardial infarction leading to cardiogenic shock

A2.

An intravenous fluid bolus of 500 ml is administered to correct hypovolaemia, in the absence of pulmonary oedema.

A3.

The provision of inotropic support is the next step: noradrenaline or dobutamine are most commonly used (although others are also available). A noradrenaline infusion via central access (4 mg of noradrenaline in 50 ml of normal saline) at a rate of 5 ml/hr is a good starting point (equivalent to 6.6 mcg/minute).

The full detail of the pathophysiology of cardiogenic shock is complex. However, to cover it briefly, ischaemia significantly depresses the contractility of the myocardium and this leads to reduced cardiac index and hypotension, which then causes even worse coronary perfusion. A reduced cardiac index results in tissue hypoperfusion (lactate is a sensitive measure of this); this cycle continues and results in death unless treatment is received. Further contributing factors include systemic inflammation, causing leaky capillaries, poor microcirculation, and vasodilatation (initial vasoconstriction as compensation is overridden).

Further Reading

Thiele H, Ohman EM, Desch S, Eitel I, de Waha S. Management of cardiogenic shock. *European Heart Journal.* 2015;36(20):1223–30.

SAQ 10 **Abnormal Computed Tomography (CT) Scan**

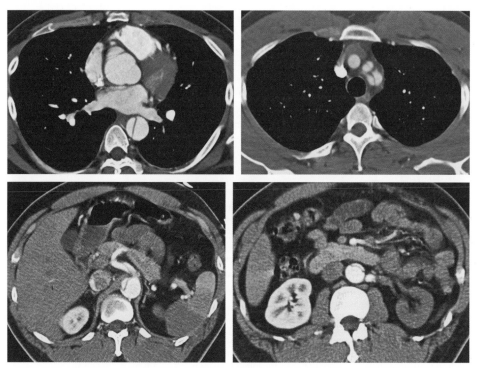

Fig. 2.7 Reproduced from Bhalla, S. et al., (2012). *Chest Imaging Cases*. Oxford: Oxford University Press. Copyright © 2012 by Oxford University Press, Inc. Reproduced with permission of the Licensor through PLSclear.

Q1. This patient presents with chest pain. Describe the CT abnormality in Fig. 2.7. What is the diagnosis?

Q2. Describe a classification system for this condition.

Q3. List the options available for medical management.

Answers

A1.

There is a double lumen in the aorta caused by an intimal flap, the diagnosis is thoracic aortic dissection.

The classic patient is an older male (aged 70 years or more), with hypertension and acute onset chest pain. Indeed, over two-thirds of patients with aortic dissection have a history of hypertension. Medical school teaching suggests that chest pain is of a 'tearing/ripping' nature, however, this is not what characteristically happens in clinical practice. A 'sharp' pain is much more commonly described. The idea of a migratory pattern of pain is reported in a minority of patients. Some patients do present without pain and their presenting symptom is syncope. This indicates that clinical examination is key to identifying other suspicious features such as pulse deficit and an aortic regurgitation murmur. Chest radiography, while useful in some patients, can be falsely reassuring if there is no evidence of mediastinal widening or unusual aortic shape.

A2.

Classification systems for aortic dissection include one of:

- De Bakey
    Type I—Originates in ascending aorta, propagates at least to the aortic arch
    Type II—Originates in ascending aorta and is confined to the ascending aorta.
    Type III—Originates in descending aorta, rarely extends proximally but will extend distally
- Stanford

    A—Involves the ascending aorta and/or aortic arch, and possibly the descending aorta. The tear can originate in the ascending aorta, the aortic arch, or, more rarely, in the descending aorta.
    B—Involves the descending aorta or the arch (distal to the left subclavian artery), without involvement of the ascending aorta.
Generally, the Stanford classification is preferred.

A3.

Medical management is often appropriate for initial management of a type B dissection.

The target blood pressure is less than 120/80 mm Hg and target heart rate less than 60 beats per minute, provided that urine output and other indicators of end-organ perfusion are maintained.

The first-choice agent is therefore a beta-receptor antagonist: an intravenous bolus and infusion of esmolol, propranolol, or labetalol is given. After adequate beta-blockade is achieved, adjunctive intravenous sodium nitroprusside can be added. If myocardial ischaemia is present, intravenous glyceryl trinitrate is a good choice for additional blood pressure lowering.

Further Reading

Hagan PG, Nienaber CA, Isselbacher EM, Bruckman D, Karavite DJ, Russman PL, et al. The International Registry of Acute Aortic Dissection (IRAD): new insights into an old disease. *Journal of the American Medical Association*. 2000;283(7):897–903.

SAQ 11 **Collapse in a Young Person**

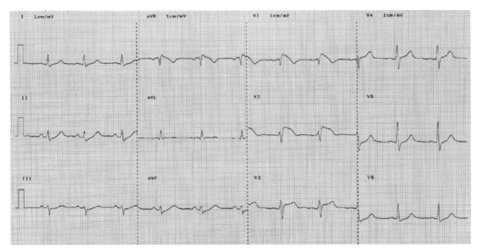

Fig. 2.8 Reproduced from Myerson, S., Choudhury, R. and Mitchell, A. (2010). *Emergencies in Cardiology*. 2nd ed. Oxford: Oxford University Press. © Oxford University Press 2009. Reproduced with permission of the Licensor through PLSclear.

A 22-year-old male presents after a collapse while at university. The ECG shown in Fig. 2.8 is obtained. He has no past medical history but tells you that his brother died unexpectedly at the age of 18 years.

Q1. What are the abnormalities on the ECG?

Q2. What is the diagnosis?

Q3. What is the definite long-term management required for these patients?

Answers

A1.

The ECG shows coved ST segment elevation in aVR, V1, and V2.

A2.

The diagnosis is Brugada syndrome.

NB: These ECG changes are suggestive but not diagnostic of Brugada syndrome. There are three types of Brugada syndrome, and the ECG changes can be transient.

A3.

As there is a risk of ventricular tachyarrhythmia and potential sudden cardiac death, an ICD is required.

Brugada syndrome is autosomal dominant and leads to sudden cardiac death associated with one of multiple ECG patterns which span incomplete right bundle branch block and ST elevation in the anterior chest leads. These patients develop ventricular tachyarrhythmia which may then lead to syncope, cardiac arrest, and subsequent death. There are eight different genes with mutations known to cause this syndrome. Currently treatment involves placement of an automatic ICD which can prevent death by managing ventricular tachycardia or fibrillation. Use of medications such as isoprenaline or quinidine is very limited. The former can be used to treat electrical storm and the latter is used in those with ICDs following multiple shocks, those in whom an implantable ICD is contraindicated, and in those who develop supraventricular tachycardia.

Further Reading

Sheikh AS, Ranjan K. Brugada syndrome: a review of the literature. *Clinical Medicine (London)*. 2014;4(5):482–9.

SAQ 12 **Palpitations**

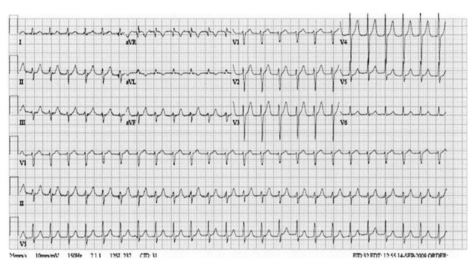

Fig. 2.9 Reproduced from Gray, R. and Pack, L. (2011). *Cardiovascular Disease in the Elderly*. Oxford: Oxford University Press. © Oxford University Press, 2011. Reproduced with permission of the Licensor through PLSclear.

A 50-year-old lady presents with an acute onset of palpitations. Her ECG is seen in Fig. 2.9.

Q1. What is the diagnosis in Fig. 2.9?

Q2. List three adverse features associated with this condition.

Q3. What is the first-line drug therapy and what might contraindicate this?

Answers

A1.

The diagnosis is atrioventricular nodal re-entrant tachycardia (AVNRT), which is the most common form of supraventricular tachycardia. It is described as a re-entrant tachycardia which involves two functionally discrete pathways usually denoted 'fast' and 'slow'. Other variants are recorded, such as 'slow-slow'. Slow-fast AVNRT (with a slow anterograde atrioventricular (AV) nodal pathway and a fast retrograde AV nodal pathway) typically presents as a regular narrow complex tachycardia, with absent P waves and small pseudo r' waves (representing retrograde P waves) in V1, and occasionally in leads II, III, and aVF. Normally it is seen in young people without any structural heart condition or ischaemic heart disease. Almost two-thirds of cases are seen in females. The ventricular rate is frequently between 180 and 200 beats per minute, but can be over 250 and very occasionally under 100.

A2.

Adverse features associated with AVNRT include three from:

- Syncope
- Ischaemic chest pain
- Heart failure
- Systolic blood pressure below 90 mm Hg

A3.

Adenosine 6 mg/12 mg/12 mg rapid intravenous bolus injections, followed by a 20 ml saline flush; repeated at one-minute intervals, would constitute first-line therapy. It would be contraindicated by asthma, chronic obstructive pulmonary disease (COPD), and second- or third-degree atrioventricular block. Second-line options include a beta-blocker if left ventricular function is not impaired (e.g. intravenous metoprolol 5 mg, or a calcium channel blocker, e.g. intravenous verapamil 5–10 mg over 30 seconds). If you do give adenosine and the patient becomes dyspnoeic and wheezy, you can consider using 50–250 mg intravenous aminophylline over 30–60 seconds to antagonize the theophylline.

Before initiating drug therapy, vagotonic manoeuvres such as carotid sinus massage (5 seconds), a Valsalva manoeuvre-expiration against a closed glottis (10–15 seconds) or Muller manoeuvre-sudden inspiration against a closed glottis, can be attempted.

Further Reading

Page RL, Joglar JA, Caldwell MA, Calkins H, Conti JB, Deal BJ, et al. (2016). 2015 ACC/AHA/HRS Guideline for the Management of Adult Patients with Supraventricular Tachycardia: Executive Summary: A report of the American College of Cardiology/American Heart Association Task Force on Clinical Practice Guidelines and the Heart Rhythm Society. *Journal of the American College of Cardiology.* 2016;67(13):1575–623.

SAQ 13 **Abnormal ECG 2**

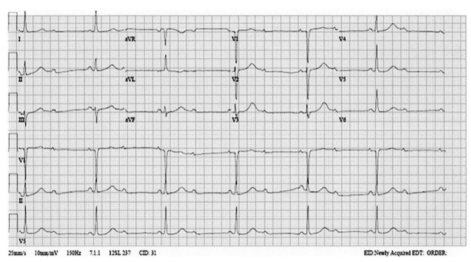

Fig. 2.10 Reproduced from Gray, R. and Pack, L. (2011). *Cardiovascular Disease in the Elderly*. Oxford: Oxford University Press. © Oxford University Press, 2011. Reproduced with permission of the Licensor through PLSclear.

The triage nurse shows you this ECG in Fig. 2.10.

Q1. What is the diagnosis?
Q2. List two systemic conditions that can precipitate this.
Q3. You call the cardiology team. What is their advice?

Answers

A1.

The diagnosis is second-degree heart block, Mobitz type 2, 2:1.

   Usually the causative lesion lies within the atrioventricular node or the His-Purkinje system. In 2:1 atrioventricular block we see only one conducted P wave for every P wave which has been blocked. In a 2:1 AV block, there is only one conducted P wave for each P wave blocked. A 2:1 block with bundle branch block is an indication of infranodal block and therefore a pacemaker is often indicated even if the patient is asymptomatic. However, if the block is found to be in the atrioventricular node, then this may not be the case.

A2.

Systemic causes include two from:

- Sarcoidosis
- Hyperkalaemia
- Amyloidosis
- Systemic lupus erythematosus

A3.

Mobitz type 2 second-degree AV block is much more likely than Mobitz type 1 to be associated with haemodynamic compromise, severe bradycardia, and progression to third-degree heart block. Onset of haemodynamic instability may be sudden and unexpected, causing syncope (Stokes–Adams attacks) or sudden cardiac death. The risk of asystole is around 35% per year. The presence of Mobitz type 2 block mandates immediate admission for cardiac monitoring, backup temporary pacing, followed by insertion of a permanent pacemaker.

Further Reading

Barold SS, Hayes DL. Second-degree atrioventricular block: a reappraisal. *Mayo Clinic Proceedings* 2001;76(1):44–57.

SAQ 14 **Dyspnoea**

An 85-year-old man presents with increasing shortness of breath and is noted to have pitting ankle and leg oedema. You obtain a chest radiograph as part of your diagnostic workup (see Fig. 2.11).

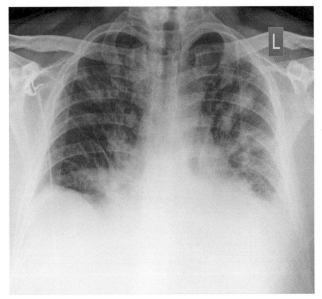

Fig. 2.11 Reproduced from Tubaro, M. et al. (2015). *The ESC Textbook of Intensive and Acute Cardiovascular Care.* 2nd ed. Oxford: Oxford University Press. © European Society of Caridology, 2015. Reproduced with permission of the Licensor through PLSclear.

Q1.   What is the diagnosis based on the presentation and the chest X-ray shown in Fig. 2.11?

Q2.   What treatment will you start in the emergency department?

Q3.   What is the role of point-of-care ultrasound in this condition?

Answers

A1.

The diagnosis is acute pulmonary oedema. Chest radiographs of pulmonary oedema may show blunting of the costophrenic angles, upper lobe diversion, Kerley B lines, and pleural effusions.

A2.

Besides high flow oxygen and intravenous diuretics, the main stay of treatment is to start vasodilation (blood pressure permitting): start a glyceryl trinitrate (GTN) infusion (50 mg in 50 ml N saline) at rate of 1–10 ml/hr keeping the blood pressure above 100 mm Hg systolic. If this fails, continuous positive airway pressure (CPAP) support can be used.

A3.

One can look for signs of pulmonary congestion (sonographic B lines, which equate to Kerley B lines on plain chest films and are often picked up at an earlier stage than changes are detectable on radiographs), signs of volume overload (diameter and collapsibility of the IVC), and also evaluate left ventricular function by measurement of the ejection fraction.

The causes of heart failure can be split into:

- Myocardial disease (such as ischaemic heart disease, toxic damage, immune-mediated/ inflammatory change, metabolic derangement, and genetic abnormalities)
- Abnormal loading conditions (such as hypertension, valvular/structural defects, pericardial/ epicardial pathology, high output states, and volume overload)
- Arrhythmias (divided into tachyarrhythmias and bradyarrhythmias)

Further Reading

Ponikowski P, Voors AA, Anker SD, Bueno H, Cleland JG, Coats AJ, et al. 2016 ESC Guidelines for the diagnosis and treatment of acute and chronic heart failure: the Task Force for the diagnosis and treatment of acute and chronic heart failure of the European Society of Cardiology (ESC)Developed with the special contribution of the Heart Failure Association (HFA) of the ESC. *European Heart Journal.* 2016;37(27):2129–200.

SAQ 15 **Elderly Unwell**

An elderly man presents to your department with nausea and vomiting, some blurring of vision, palpitations, and confusion. He recalls that he takes some medicine for his heart but is not sure what or why.

Q1. What cardioactive drug could account for his symptoms?
Q2. What biochemical abnormality is often seen in combination with this?
Q3. List three aggravating factors.

Answers

A1.

The likely diagnosis is digoxin therapy leading to toxicity. A therapeutic digoxin effect is associated with ST-segment depression resembling a 'reversed tick', and shortening of the QT interval, and may not indicate toxicity in isolation. T-wave inversion and arrhythmias indicate toxicity.

Arrhythmias associated with digoxin toxicity include multiple ventricular ectopic beats, sinus bradycardia, atrial fibrillation with a slow ventricular rate, atrioventricular block, atrial tachycardia with atrioventricular block, and bi-directional ventricular tachycardia.

A2.

Hyperkalaemia is often associated with digoxin toxicity.

A3.

Digoxin toxicity can be aggravated by hypokalaemia and by co-administration of certain drugs (calcium channel blockers, antiarrhythmic agents, diuretics, and antibiotics)

Digoxin toxicity presents with gastrointestinal (nausea, anorexia, vomiting, abdominal pain, and diarrhoea), cardiac (palpitations, syncope), visual (blurring of vision, distorted colour vision, and haloes around lights), and central nervous system (CNS) symptoms (headache, drowsiness, dizziness, confusion). A high index of suspicion is required because of the low therapeutic index. Toxicity occurs at levels above 2 ng/ml.

In digoxin overdose, its cardiac glycoside action of inhibition of sodium-potassium ATPase often results in hyperkalaemia. There were animal studies to show that with very high calcium concentrations the digoxin toxicity increases and the cardiac muscle could be placed in a non-contractile state: a 'stone-heart'. This has led to calcium being branded as contraindicated in hyperkalaemia associated with digoxin toxicity. However, a more recent retrospective study has questioned the clinical applicability of this, finding no association between the administration of intravenous calcium to treat hyperkalaemia in a digoxin toxic patient and the development of fatal dysrhythmia or increased mortality.

Further Reading

Levine M, Nikkanen H, Pallin DJ. The effects of intravenous calcium in patients with digoxin toxicity. *Journal of Emergency Medicine*. 2011;40(1):41–6.

SAQ 16 **Syncope**

A 25-year-old female has collapsed while standing at a bus stop, followed by loss of consciousness lasting under a minute. She has recovered completely and is alert, with stable vital signs, on arrival in the emergency department.

Q1. List some features that help differentiate syncope from seizure.
Q2. What abnormalities on 12-lead ECG would be relevant to the presentation? List four
Q3. How would you stratify risk in a patient with syncope?

Answers

A1.

Features which may differentiate syncope from a seizure include:

- Lateral tongue biting (pathognomonic of seizure) as opposed to a bite of the tongue tip
- Identifiable provoking factor (seen with syncope)
- Prodromal symptoms (seen with syncope)
- Post-episode confusion and drowsiness (seen with seizure)

A2.

Some 12-lead ECG abnormalities that can indicate the cause of syncope include:

- Complete (third-degree) atrioventricular block
- Mobitz type 2 second-degree atrioventricular block
- Long QT syndrome (QTc >440–450 msec in men or >460 msec in women)
- Wolff-Parkinson-White syndrome (pre-excitation syndrome)
- Hypertrophic cardiomyopathy (left ventricular hypertrophy with repolarization changes)
- Brugada syndrome (right bundle branch block with ST elevation in V1–V3)
- ECG signs of myocardial ischaemia

A3.

Risk stratification can be achieved by noting the following indicators of increased risk of a poor outcome:

- History of congestive heart failure
- Haematocrit less than 30%
- Abnormal ECG
- Shortness of breath
- Systolic blood pressure less than 90 mm Hg

(These form part of the San Francisco Syncope Rule, the acronym CHESS being a means of remembering the individual components.)

Further Reading

Brignole, M, Moya, A, de Lange, FJ,et al. 2018 ESC Guidelines *European Heart Journal*. 2018, 39(21): 1883–1948.

Chapter 3 **Care of the Elderly**

SAQ 1 **Pressure Ulcer**

A 92-year-old lady has been sent into the emergency department from a nursing home. There is no accompanying letter or staff and the ambulance sheet states that she has dementia and seems more drowsy than usual. Your nursing colleagues have undressed the lady and put her into a gown, discovering that she has two pressure ulcers: one on her right hip over her greater trochanter and the other on her right heel. There is redness with some skin loss and blistering to the former and erythema with intact skin to the latter.

Q1. During your assessment and investigation, which three features would indicate a need for systemic antibiotic treatment?

Q2. Which category(ies) of pressure ulcer does this lady have?

Q3. List three risk factors for developing a pressure ulcer.

Answers

A1.

Systemic antibiotic treatment is indicated in the following circumstances:

- Any clinical evidence of systemic sepsis
- Signs of spreading cellulitis
- Evidence of underlying osteomyelitis

A2.

This lady has pressure ulcers of category II and I, respectively.

The NPUAP/EPUAP International Pressure Ulcer Classification system is summarized as:

Category/Stage I: Non-blanchable redness of intact skin
Category/Stage II: Partial thickness skin loss or blister
Category/Stage III: Full thickness skin loss (fat visible)
Category/Stage IV: Full thickness tissue loss (muscle/bone visible)

Data from National Pressure Ulcer Advisory Panel, European Pressure Ulcer Advisory Panel and Pan Pacific Pressure Injury Alliance. *Prevention and Treatment of Pressure Ulcers: Quick Reference Guide.* Emily Haesler (Ed.). Cambridge Media: Perth, Australia; 2014.

A3.

Risk factors for developing a pressure ulcer include:

- Significantly limited mobility (e.g. people with a spinal cord injury)
- Significant loss of sensation
- A previous or current pressure ulcer
- Nutritional deficiency
- The inability to reposition themselves
- Significant cognitive impairment

Management of pressure ulcers can involve some/all of the following:

- Ulcer measurement: this may involve tracing and photography and needs an estimated depth and documented evidence of undermining.
- Categorization: as exemplified here, each ulcer must be categorized.
- Nutrition and hydration: a dietitian (or others qualified) needs to assess requirements, and support must be given to care-givers to maintain adequate nutrition. Overhydration is not beneficial therefore no subcutaneous/intravenous fluids should be given to those adequately hydrated.
- Pressure redistribution: appropriate mattresses/seat cushions must be sourced, depending on the amount of time spent lying/sitting.
- Negative pressure wound management: this should only be offered if it will reduce the number of dressing changes in such wounds with, for example, a large exudate.
- Debridement: autolytic and sharp debridement may be required, and larval therapy may also be required if sharp debridement is contraindicated or there is vascular insufficiency.
- Antibiotics: if cellulitis/systemic sepsis/osteomyelitis is present, then systemic antibiotics are required. Positive wound cultures alone are not an indication.
- Dressings: warm, moist wound dressings are recommended for grade 2–4 ulcers; however, choice of dressing also depends on tolerance, position, exudate, and frequency of changes needed. Gauze is not an appropriate choice.

Further Reading

European Pressure Ulcer Advisory Panel and National Pressure Ulcer Advisory Panel. Treatment of pressure ulcers: Quick Reference Guide. Washington DC: National Pressure Ulcer Advisory Panel; 2009.

NICE. *Pressure Ulcers: Prevention and Management CG179*. 2014. Available from: https://www.nice.org.uk/guidance/cg179/chapter/1-recommendations#management-adults

SAQ 2 **Elder Abuse**

A 92-year-old male has been brought to the emergency department following a fall. At initial assessment, he is noted to be unkempt, malnourished, and has multiple bruises of different ages.

Q1. List four types of elder abuse.
Q2. In this patient, what measures should be taken in his best interests?
Q3. List four risk factors for elder abuse.

Answers

A1.

Types of elder abuse include (choose four):

- Physical abuse
- Sexual abuse
- Emotional abuse
- Financial/material exploitation
- Neglect
- Self-neglect
- Abandonment (violation of rights)

A2.

Multiagency safeguarding referral is indicated.

There is an Action on Elder Abuse helpline (080 8808 8141) for England, Wales, Scotland, and Northern Ireland.

A3.

Risk factors for elder abuse include (choose four):

- Frailty
- Advanced age
- Female sex
- Cognitive impairment
- Mental health problems
- Social isolation of the victim
- Recent life stress

Further Reading

Dong XQ. Elder abuse: systematic review and implications for practice. *Journal of American Geriatrics Society.* 2015;63(6):1214–38.

SAQ 3 **Reduced Mobility**

An 87-year-old female, living alone in her own house, has been brought to the emergency department having 'gone off her legs'.

Q1. Considering that 7% of people report functional dependence with one health condition, what percentage report functional dependence with four health conditions?
Q2. List four other types of impairment than mobility/gait which might progressively decline.
Q3. What complications may occur as a result of immobility in older people?

Answers

A1.

Around 60%. This is important to consider when dealing with elderly patients who have multiple comorbidities, as the interaction between various health conditions means that the subsequent functional impact from having subsequent health problems is not linear.

A2.

Progressive decline may occur in (choose four):

* Cognition
* Mood
* Sensory impairment
* Pain
* Nutrition
* Medication adverse effects

A3.

Complications of immobility in older people include (choose four):

* Pressure sores
* Bone resorption; hypercalcaemia
* Atelectasis; pneumonia
* Thromboembolism
* Urine incontinence
* Constipation and faecal impaction
* Depression and anxiety

In the assessment of specific neuromusculoskeletal impairments, the following tests may be useful:

* Clasping hands behind the head and back—this identifies limitations in dressing/grooming/bathing/housework
* Placing ankle on opposite knee—this identifies limitations in dressing the lower body/bathing/toileting

- Standing from a chair without using arms—this identifies limitations in bathing/toileting and likelihood of falls
- Rise on toes (bilateral or unilateral)—this identifies limitations in stair climbing/housework/ bathing and likelihood of falls
- Gentle nudging to sternum—this identifies limitations in housework/bathing and likelihood of falls
- Standing from a chair without using arms, walking 10 feet, returning, and sitting down—this identifies limitations in mobility/bathing/toileting/housework
- Picking up a penny from the floor—this identifies limitations in cooking/feeding/grooming/ dressing/housework
- Two-minute walking distance—this identifies limitations in community mobility/shopping

There are other tests for sensory and cognitive impairment which are useful at picking up issues with social functioning, medication management, telephone use, driving, memory, activities of daily living, balance, and financial management.

These tests must also be considered in association with contextual factors, such as:

- Difficulty with stairs in and out of the home
- Confidence bathing/toileting
- Social support in the event of illness or an emergency
- Care-giving
- Nutrition maintenance

Further Reading

Colón-Emeric CS, Whitson HE, Pavon J, Hoenig H. Functional decline in older adults. *American Family Physician.* 2013;88(6):388–94.

SAQ 4 **Delirium**

A 92-year-old female has been brought to the emergency department from a residential care home as she has been increasingly confused and aggressive over the preceding two days.

Q1. List three features suggestive of delirium.
Q2. List three indications for computed tomography (CT) scan of the head.
Q3. With a restless and agitated patient, what pharmacological treatment could help facilitate a CT head scan?

Answers

A1.

Features indicative of delirium include (choose three):

- Acute onset
- Clouding of consciousness
- Fluctuating level of consciousness
- Cognitive deficits, including disorientation and impaired memory
- Altered sleep–wake cycle
- Altered arousal (hyperactive, hypoactive, or mixed forms)
- Impaired attention
- Visual or auditory hallucinations

A2.

The indications for CT head scan include:

- History of head injury
- Depressed level of consciousness
- Focal neurological findings
- Evidence of raised intracranial pressure

A3.

A small dose of lorazepam or low dose haloperidol (0.5–1 mg oral or intramuscular) may be considered to facilitate cooperation with imaging. Antipsychotic medication can be complicated by extrapyramidal side effects, and benzodiazepines can cause excessive sedation, paradoxical excitation, and respiratory depression.

It is important to consider delirium in those at higher risk of developing it such as:

- Those over 65
- Those with pre-existing cognitive impairment
- Currently fractured hip
- Severe illness (i.e. a condition which is getting worse or has the potential to get worse)

Prevention of delirium can begin in the emergency department by taking the following steps:

- Try to maintain the same care personnel and environment to promote familiarity
- Assess possible risk factors for delirium
- Ensure clocks and calendars are available
- Check regularly where the person is, why they are there, and who is caring for them
- Provide some cognitive stimulation
- Ensure family and friends are able to visit
- Monitor for evidence of dehydration and managing this
- Maintain regular bowel movements
- Avoid hypoxia
- Manage any evidence of infection
- Avoid unnecessary catheterization
- Encourage mobilization at the earliest opportunity
- Manage pain (and look out for non-verbal cues)
- Review medication to ensure contributory medications are avoided where possible
- Maintain good nutrition
- Address any hearing aid requirements/wax impaction
- Ensure spectacles are available for those needing them
- Promote good sleep (although this is easier in a ward environment)

Further Reading

NICE (2014). *Delirium in adults*, QS63. Available from: https://www.nice.org.uk

SAQ 5 **Fall with Prolonged Lie**

A 92-year-old female has been found by her carer at home, lying on the floor in a corridor at 8 am, and has been sent to the emergency department. She was last seen at 6 pm the previous day. She was unable to get up, and it is thought she may have fallen at around 10 pm on the way to the toilet.

Q1. List three potential complications after a prolonged lie following a fall.
Q2. List three investigations that are indicated.
Q3. What specific management is indicated? List three options.

Answers

A1.

Complications of a prolonged lie following a fall include (choose three):

- Dehydration
- Pressure sores
- Carpet burns
- Skeletal injuries
- Rhabdomyolysis
- Acute kidney injury
- Hypothermia
- Pneumonia

A2.

Investigations that are relevant to this situation include (choose three):

- Urea and electrolytes: this may show high potassium, low calcium, and high phosphate
- Serum creatine kinase: a rise of five times baseline or greater is diagnostic for rhabdomyolysis
- Urine dipstick: myoglobin may cause a positive test for blood; there may be evidence of a urinary tract infection, necessitating getting up at night to pass urine
- Chest X-ray: may show rib fractures, or evidence of pneumonia
- Plain X-rays for suspected fractures based on clinical assessment, such as pelvis, humerus, wrist, cervical spine
- 12-lead electrocardiogram (ECG)

A3.

Interventions that may need to be commenced in the emergency department include (choose three):

- Rehydration, especially with a high serum creatine kinase
- Rewarming for hypothermia
- Pressure area care
- Functional assessment (e.g. occupational therapy) if no immediate need for hospitalization and treatment

When a patient is admitted it is very important that risk factors for fall in hospital are identified in order that they can be managed appropriately. These risk factors may include:

- Cognitive impairment
- Problems of incontinence
- Any history of falls (this includes causes and consequences of such, e.g. injury or fear of falling)
- Footwear which is unsuitable or simply missing
- Health issues
- Medications
- Postural instability
- Mobility
- Balance problems
- Syncopal episodes
- Visual impairment

(Source: Falls in older people QS86, NICE, 2015)

Chapter 4 Critical Care and Anaesthesia

SAQ 1 **Rapid Sequence Induction**

Your trainees are keen for a teaching session and refresher on the principles of rapid sequence induction (RSI) having all done their anaesthetics attachment over a year ago. They have a few questions during the session:

Q1. In any RSI scenario what is the maximum number of attempts at intubation that should be made (according to guidance) before plan B of the anaesthetic plan should be followed?

Q2. What are the benefits of rocuronium over suxamethonium in RSI?

Q3. What effect does cricoid pressure have on the use of supraglottic airway devices?

Answers

A1.

Three attempts by one, followed possibly by one further attempt by a more experienced colleague.
    (Taken from the Difficult Airway Society's 'Intubation guidelines—Rapid sequence induction')

A2.

Rocuronium can be reversed by sugammadex, administered as a single intravenous bolus over 10 seconds. Rocuronium does not cause oxygen-consuming fasciculations in the same way suxamethonium does.

Suxamethonium is the agent traditionally used due to speed of onset negating bag-valve ventilation. However, studies suggest that overall, the use of rocuronium is comparable. The oxygen consumption generated by fasciculations may overall make suxamethonium less favourable in the event of airway obstruction. Suxamethonium cannot be antagonized in the same way rocuronium can be, however, this antagonism does not guarantee a patent airway. If rocuronium is used, then the correct dose of sugammadex must be available immediately (16 mg/kg).

A3.

Cricoid pressure reduces hypopharyngeal space so it should not be used when using supraglottic airway devices.

It is interesting that cricoid pressure is an integral part of the rapid sequence induction procedure, commonly assumed to be preventative of reflux of gastric contents and improved laryngoscopic view, when in fact the original purpose of this technique was described as preventing gastric distension during mask ventilation. Being able to gently ventilate using a mask is a useful technique to prolong time to desaturation, especially in those with sepsis, poor respiratory reserve, and high metabolic requirements.

One notable potential pitfall of cricoid pressure is that it can reduce lower oesophageal sphincter tone and thus regurgitation may become more likely.

The referenced article gives a good overview of difficult airway management (which is a term that applies to all patients being considered for RSI in the emergency department).

Further Reading

Frerk C, Mitchell VS, McNarry AF, Mendonca C, Bhagrath R, Patel A, et al. Difficult Airway Society 2015 guidelines for management of unanticipated difficult intubation in adults. *British Journal of Anaesthesia*. 2015;115(6):827–48.

SAQ 2 **Propofol**

Your higher specialty training (ST3) trainees are keen to get some experience in conscious sedation following from their anaesthetic placement the preceding year. They are very keen to use propofol as they have seen the anaesthetists use it frequently; you are keen that they understand a bit more about the drug so they can use it safely. You consider some questions for a teaching session.

Q1. What is the mechanism of action of propofol?
Q2. What is its main advantage in the emergency department?
Q3. What is a common complaint of patients receiving propofol?

Answers

A1.

Propofol reduces the rate of gamma-aminobutyric acid (GABA) dissociation from GABA receptors, which increases the opening time of the GABA-activated chloride channel that results in the cell membrane being hyperpolarized. At high enough concentrations, it may independently activate the GABA-receptor's chloride channel. This action increases GABA-mediated inhibitory tone in the central nervous system.

A2.

The main advantage of propofol in the emergency setting is its rapid onset of action and recovery time. The onset of action is within 15–45 seconds of administration, leading to loss of consciousness with one arm–brain circulation time). The redistribution half-life of 1–3 minutes leads to cessation of effect after a single dose.

A3.

Propofol causes pain on injection. This can be mitigated by the administration of very small amounts of intravenous local anaesthetic.

Further Reading

Trapani G, Altomare C, Liso G, Sanna E, Biggio G. Propofol in anesthesia. Mechanism of action, structure-activity relationships, and drug delivery. *Current Medicinal Chemistry*. 2000;7(2):249–71.

SAQ 3 **Fascia Iliaca Block**

An 87-year-old lady has fallen in her nursing home and has sustained a fractured neck of right femur. You decide she needs a fascia iliaca block for pain relief.

Q1. Give at least three indications for a fascia iliaca compartment block.

Q2. Label Fig. 4.1 with the femoral nerve and the fascia iliaca.

Q3. Describe the approach and technique for performing an ultrasound guided fascia iliaca block.

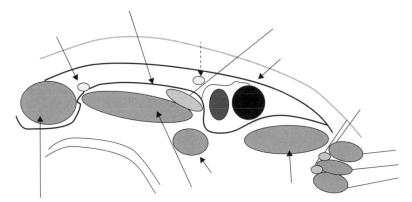

Fig. 4.1 Adapted with permission from Range C, Egeler C. Fascia. Iliaca Compartment Block: Landmark and Ultrasound Approach. Anaesthesia Tutorial of the Week [Internet]. 2010. Available from: http://www.frca. co.uk/Documents/193%20Fascia%20Iliaca%20compartment%20block.pdf

---

Answers

A1.

Indications for fascia iliaca block include (three from):

- Perioperative analgesia for fractured neck/shaft of the femur
- Additional analgesia during hip surgery
- Analgesia for above-knee amputations
- Analgesia for applying plaster to children with a fractured femur
- Analgesia when combined with a sciatic nerve block for knee operations
- Analgesia to cover pain from lower leg tourniquet during awake operations

A2.

See Fig. 4.2 for a labelled image.

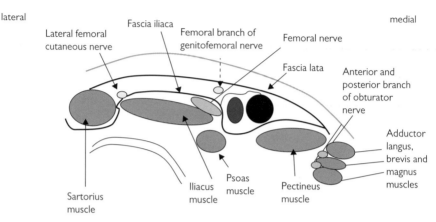

Fig. 4.2 Adapted with permission from Range C, Egeler C. Fascia. Iliaca Compartment Block: Landmark and Ultrasound Approach. Anaesthesia Tutorial of the Week [Internet]. 2010. Available from: http://www.frca. co.uk/Documents/193%20Fascia%20Iliaca%20compartment%20block.pdf

A3.

The technique includes the following steps:

- Make usual aseptic no-touch technique preparations and gather all equipment and local anaesthetic
- Place the high frequency ultrasound probe in a horizontal plane just distal to the inguinal ligament
- Try to orientate yourself to the location of the femoral artery and the iliacus muscle, which is lateral to it and covered by the fascia iliaca
- If the femoral artery is seen to divide, move the probe more cranially
- Advance the needle tip from a lateral to medial direction (either in or out of plane)
- Place the tip beneath the fascia iliaca, trying to feel as the fascia lata is first breached and then the fascia iliaca
- Confirm no blood can be aspirated before every local anaesthetic injection
- The flow of anaesthetic should be easy and if resistance is felt, it may be within the iliacus muscle—withdrawal of the needle a little may help
- Spread of the injected fluid should be seen to separate the planes on ultrasound, spreading the fascia iliaca compartment

Further Reading

Range C, Egeler C. *Fascia Iliaca Compartment Block: Landmark and Ultrasound Approach—Anaesthesia Tutorial of the Week*. 2010. Available from: http://www.frca.co.uk/Documents/193%20Fascia%20Iliaca%20compartment%20block.pdf

SAQ 4 **Intraosseous Needle**

You are part of a team dealing with a two-year-old child presenting with septic shock in the resuscitation room. Several attempts at obtaining peripheral venous access have failed. You ask for an intraosseous needle set.

Q1. List three contraindications for an intraosseous needle.
Q2. What sites are suitable for introduction of the needle in this child?
Q3. Mention two complications of the procedure.

Answers

A1.

Contraindications to intraosseous needle placement include (three from):

- Fracture in the selected bone
- Local infection such as cellulitis
- Clotting disorder
- Osteogenesis imperfecta

A2.

Suitable sites for introduction of an intraosseous needle include:

- Proximal tibia (anteromedial surface)
- Distal femur (anterolateral surface)
- The proximal humerus is an option in children aged 5 years or above

A3.

Complications include (two from):

- Infection
- Extravasation of infused fluid
- Fracture of the bone or physeal plate
- Compartment syndrome

Interosseous needles are invaluable in the administration of emergency fluids and medications; these can be delivered at similar rates to intravenous and central routes. Pressure infusion bags do help to improve flow rates when used with adult needles. Although many sites have potential for intraosseous access (proximal tibia, distal tibia, sternum, radius, clavicle, proximal humerus, and calcaneum), ideally the site should be a large long bone, have easily identifiable landmarks, be superficial, be easily accessible percutaneously, and be relatively proximal to ensure medications and fluids reach the central circulation quickly. Furthermore, ideally the site needs to be away from areas which are in the way of the resuscitation effort and which cannot easily cause damage to nearby structures if accidentally knocked. As such this makes sternal and clavicular sites unfavourable. Similarly, distal tibia, radius, and calcaneum are considered too distal.

Further Reading

Ngo AS, Oh JJ, Chen Y, Yong D, Ong ME. Intraosseous vascular access in adults using the EZ-IO in an emergency department. *International Journal of Emergency Medicine*. 2009;2(3):155–60.

SAQ 5 **Procedural Sedation**

You have been asked to provide procedural sedation for a 40-year-old female brought to the resuscitation room with an ankle dislocation.

Q1. List four qualities of an ideal sedative.
Q2. What is the mechanism by which ketamine works?
Q3. What aspects make up an appropriate airway assessment?

Answers

A1.

The following qualities would be exhibited by an ideal sedative:

- Sedation, with a dose-dependent depression of level of consciousness which is easily titratable
- Anxiolysis
- Amnesia
- Analgesia
- Rapid onset and offset of action, with inactive metabolites
- Short-acting; reversibility of action
- No accumulation in the presence of renal or hepatic impairment
- Minimal side effects, such as haemodynamic impairment, respiratory depression, or uncontrolled movements
- No or minimal interaction with other drugs

A2.

Ketamine is an NMDA (N-methyl-D-aspartate) receptor antagonist, with dissociative, hallucinogenic, and euphoria-producing properties in addition to analgesia.

A3.

Airway assessment entails the following steps:

- **L**ook—patient specific characteristics that are known to cause difficulty with intubation or ventilation
- **E**valuate—Mouth opening and thyromental distance (3-3-2 rule)
- **M**allampati score
- **O**bstruction—upper airway pathology
- **N**eck mobility

Here are some details about common sedative agents used in the emergency department:

- Entonox®: it is thought this binds to central opioid receptors and can cause side effects such as vomiting. It should not be used in those with head injury, pneumothorax, bowel obstruction, and sinus disease.
- Propofol: as a lipophilic phenol derivative it crosses the blood–brain barrier very quickly and is useful for sedation and amnesia. For sedation, even a dose such as 10 mg may be enough depending on age and comorbidity. It should be noted that while its action may be seen at 30 seconds, it may take 2 minutes for peak effect, especially in older patients. Soy and egg lecithin form part of the preparations so care should be taken with allergies.
- Midazolam: the side effects can include respiratory depression, hypotension, and— paradoxically—disinhibition and agitation in children at low doses. It does accumulate in adipose tissue which can prolong its sedative effects; similarly, in older people, the obese, or those with hepatic/renal disease it can have a prolonged effect.
- Ketamine: this is a phencyclidine derivative producing a dissociative state and profound analgesia with superficial sleep. There is no dose–response continuum. Instead there is a threshold dose for dissociation and then further doses maintain the state. At subdisassociative doses, analgesia and disorientation occur. Absolute contraindications include those below three months of age, and those with known or suspected schizophrenia. Relative contraindications include active pulmonary disease or infection, known or suspected cardiovascular disease, central nervous system masses, abnormalities, and hydrocephalus, globe injury, or glaucoma.
- Fentanyl: this has up to 125 times the potency of morphine and starts to work at around 2–3 minutes, lasting around 30–60 minutes. Those with renal/hepatic impairment and the elderly may have profound or prolonged effects.

Further Reading

RCEM. *Pharmacological Agents for Procedural Sedation and Analgesia in the Emergency Department: Best Practice Guideline*. May 2016. Available from: https://www.rcem.ac.uk/docs/College%20Guidelines/Pharmacological%20Agents%20for%20Procedural%20Sedation%20and%20Analgesia%20(Oct%202016).pdf

Chapter 5 **Dermatology**

SAQ 1 **Circular Rash**

A 23-year-old lady presents generally unwell with muscle pain. She had been hiking through Exmoor a week ago. You notice the rash in Fig. 5.1.

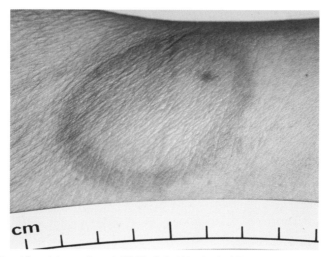

Fig. 5.1 Reproduced from Johnson, C. et al. (2015). *Oxford Handbook of Expedition and Wilderness Medicine.* 2nd ed. Oxford: Oxford University Press. © Oxford University Press 2015. Reproduced with permission of the licensor via PLSClear.

Q1. Give a typical description of and name this rash.
Q2. What is the causative organism and the diagnosis?
Q3. List three non-neurological complications.

Answers

A1.

This is an extending macular rash with central clearing and is known as erythema migrans. The rash has been likened to the bull's eye on a dart board.

A2.

The causative organism is Borrelia burgdorferi, a spirochaetal organism, causing Lyme disease.

A3.

Non-neurological complications include (three from):

- Conduction system disorder: atrioventricular nodal block—first degree/complete
- Conjunctivitis
- Optic neuropathy
- Lyme arthritis: intermittent or persistent inflammatory arthritis involving one or a few large joints, most commonly the knee joint
- Acrodermatitis chronica atrophicans

Lyme disease was first described following an outbreak in Old Lyme, Connecticut, in 1975. The incubation period ranges from 3 to 32 days after exposure to an infected tick. In Europe, the countries with highest prevalence of Lyme disease are the Netherlands, Austria, Estonia, Lithuania, and Slovenia. Erythema migrans (EM) appears at the bite site within 7 to 14 days and must be differentiated from an allergic reaction rash (tends to occur sooner). EM is often associated with a viral prodrome (myalgia, fatigue, headache). It does not lead to upper respiratory or gastrointestinal symptoms.

Late neurological complications of Lyme are nerve palsies (especially facial nerve), meningitis, and radiculopathies. Lyme disease can be treated using doxycycline, amoxicillin, or cephalosporin for 2–3 weeks. Do not prescribe doxycycline to pregnant patients as this may affect the fetus's skeletal development (if given in first trimester) or discoloured teeth (second/third trimester)

Further Reading

CDC. *Ticks and Lyme Disease.* Available from: https://www.cdc.gov/lyme/resources/toolkit/factsheets/10_508_Lyme-disease_PregnantWoman_FACTSheet.pdf

Shapiro ED. Clinical practice. Lyme disease. *New England Journal of Medicine.* 2014;370(18):1724–31.

SAQ 2 **Swelling of Lips**

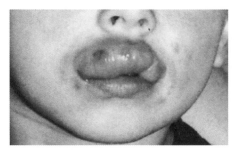

Fig. 5.2 Reproduced from Lewis-Jones, S. (2010). *Paediatric Dermatology*. Oxford University Press. © Oxford University Press 2010. Reproduced with permission of the licensor via PLSClear.

Q1. What does Fig. 5.2 show?
Q2. Give ways you might classify different causes of this condition?
Q3. How does treatment differ between different aetiologies of this condition?

Answers

A1.

Angioedema of the lips. Angioedema involves the deep dermis, subcutaneous, and submucosal tissues, as opposed to urticaria, which involves the epidermis and dermis only, and is non-pitting with pressure.

A2.

The causes can be categorized as:

- Hereditary angioedema (decreased C1 inhibitor activity)
- Acquired angioedema
- Drug-induced angioedema
- Allergic angioedema
- Idiopathic angioedema

A3.

Treatments include:

- Allergic angioedema: give antihistamines, steroids, and—if needed—intramuscular adrenaline
- ACEI-induced angioedema: replace C1 inhibitor, discontinue the drug causing oedema
- Hereditary angioedema: replace C1 inhibitor

It is important for the clinician to differentiate between histamine or bradykinin as the likely aetiology of the angioedema. Histamine-related angioedema is more commonly associated with itching, erythema, and bronchospasm. Bradykinin-related angioedema lacks these urticarial signs.

Mast cell-mediated pathologies can be successfully treated by antihistamine, steroids, and if severe (anaphylaxis), IM adrenaline. In bradykinin-mediated pathologies, antihistamines and steroid therapies are not beneficial.

Hereditary angioedema (HA) is a rare autosomal dominant disorder characterized by recurrent episodes of angioedema. ACEI (angiotensin-converting enzyme inhibitor) angioedema is a side effect of the use of ACEI and two-thirds of all episodes usually starts within 3 months of initiating therapy with an ACEI. Reports of onset after years of therapy have also been published. Treatment for both HA and ACEI angioedema include C1 inhibitor concentrate, icatibant (a bradykinin receptor antagonist), or fresh frozen plasma (FFP). FFP contains angiotensin-converting enzymes (ACE), which can help in ACEI-induced angioedema if no other products are available. ACEI angioedema requires cessation of the offending drug.

Further Reading

Cicardi M, Aberer W, Banerji A, Bas M, Bernstein JA, Bork K, et al. Classification, diagnosis, and approach to treatment for angioedema: consensus report from the Hereditary Angioedema International Working Group. *Allergy*. 2014;69(5):602–16.

Malde B, Regalado J, Greenberger PA. Investigation of angioedema associated with the use of angiotensin-converting enzyme inhibitors and angiotensin receptor blockers. *Ann Allergy Asthma Immunol*. 2007;98(1):57–63.

SAQ 3 **Itchy Rash**

You are seeing a 63-year-old male who has been working in the garden. He presents 24 hours after the onset of a red itchy skin rash on his upper limbs which developed shortly after he went indoors. He has no systemic symptoms and is otherwise fit and well. The rash appears erythematous with an irregular surface due to multiple papules and small vesicles, and there are some linear excoriations.

Q1. What is the most likely diagnosis?
Q2. What treatment measures would you consider?
Q3. What complications would you inform him about?

Answers

A1.

The most likely diagnosis is allergic or irritant contact dermatitis.

A2.

Treatment includes:

• Topical corticosteroids
• Antihistamines
• Cold compresses

A3.

Complications to be aware of include:

• Secondary bacterial infection, usually staphylococcal and streptococcal such as erysipelas
• Systemic sepsis

As the presentation of these symptoms to emergency departments is especially common in the spring and summer months, it is important to reduce an overzealous use of antibiotics. While a superimposed cellulitis is possible, the most common origin of the erythema and pain post-insect bite is a delayed IgE-based reaction. In the absence of fevers/rigors, expectant management can be initiated: withhold antibiotics, give a short course of oral steroids, and consider use of antihistamines. If infective symptoms were to occur, the patient should return to the emergency department.

Further Reading

Carlson J, Golden, D. Large local reactions to insect envenomation. *Current Opinion in Allergy & Clinical Immunology.* 2016:16(4):366–9.
Eriksson B, Jorup-Rönström C, Karkkonen K, Sjöblom AC, Holm SE. Erysipelas: clinical and bacteriologic spectrum and serological aspects. *Clinical Infectious Diseases.* 1996;23(5):1091–8.

SAQ 4 **Painful Skin Rash**

You are seeing a 37-year-old female patient, who is on antiepileptic medication. She presents with a painful and tender red skin rash consisting of macules, papules, vesicles, flaccid blisters, and urticarial plaques. The rash is associated with purulent conjunctivitis and stomatitis.

Q1. What is the most likely diagnosis?
Q2. List three management priorities
Q3. What is the most important differential diagnosis?

Answers

A1.

The most likely diagnosis is Stevens–Johnson syndrome (SJS).

A2.

Management priorities include (three from):

- Fluid and electrolyte replacement, which may follow burn treatment guidelines
- Withdrawal of causative medications
- Eye care: lubricating eye drops; ophthalmological consultation
- Mouth care: regular mouthwashes

A3.

The differential diagnosis includes toxic epidermal necrolysis.

   Steven–Johnson syndrome and toxic epidermal necrolysis (TEN) form a spectrum of skin disease characterized by necrosis and detachment of epidermis. SJS and TEN are differentiated by the size of the total body surface (TBS) they affect: SJS is associated with epidermal detachment involving 10% or less of the TBS area. TEN involves more than 30% of TBS area. Besides the necrosis and epidermal detachment, common findings include mucous membrane lesions (genital, mouth, or eyes). The use of certain medications is associated with SJS/TEN: allopurinol, lamotrigine, phenobarbital, and carbamazepine. Mycoplasma pneumonia has also been associated with SJS/TEN and HIV is a recognized risk factor.

   Treatment is based on stopping the offending medication and offering supportive treatment with intravenous fluids, analgesia, and standard wound management. Prophylactic antibiotics are not recommended.

Further Reading

Hazin R, Ibrahimi OA, Hazin MI, Kimyai-Asadi A. Stevens–Johnson syndrome: pathogenesis, diagnosis, and management. *Annals of Medicine.* 2008;40(2):129–38.

SAQ 5 **Lower Limb Cellulitis**

A 70-year-old female attends hospital with a spreading red skin rash of the left lower leg of two days' duration. She does not recall any preceding trauma or any previous similar episodes. She gives a past medical history of hypertension and type 2 diabetes mellitus. On examination, you make a diagnosis of cellulitis.

Q1.   What additional clinical examination should be performed? List three signs you would look for.
Q2.   What factors would determine the need for admission?
Q3.   If felt to be suitable for ambulatory treatment, what treatment would you recommend?

Answers

A1.

The following signs should be looked for (three from):

- Haemodynamic status, as judged by vital signs: signs of sepsis syndrome
- Signs of arterial insufficiency
- Signs of chronic venous insufficiency
- Lymphangitis

A2.

Admission to hospital is indicated with:

- Eron Class III (acute confusion, tachycardia, tachypnoea, hypotension, or unstable comorbidities)
- Class IV (sepsis syndrome)
- Arterial insufficiency
- Significant lymphoedema

A3.

Outpatient antibiotic therapy may involve either flucloxacillin 500 mg four times a day (QDS) orally or clarithromycin 250 mg twice a day (BD) orally.
   A classification system that can help decision whether a patient is suitable for ambulatory treatment or requires admission has been devised by Eron:

> Class I patients have no signs of systemic toxicity, have no uncontrolled co-morbidities and can usually be managed with oral antimicrobials on an outpatient basis.

> Class II patients are either systemically ill or systemically well but with a co-morbidity such as peripheral vascular disease, chronic venous insufficiency or morbid obesity which may complicate or delay resolution of their infection.

> Class III patients may have a significant systemic upset such as acute confusion, tachycardia, tachypnoea, hypotension, or may have unstable co-morbidities that may interfere with a response to therapy or have a limb threatening infection due to vascular compromise.

Class IV patients have sepsis syndrome or severe life-threatening infection such as necrotizing fasciitis.

Class II–IV require admission and FBC, CRP, U&E, skin swab. Class III–IV require blood cultures. Intravenous antibiotics effective against beta-haemolytic streptococci and *Staphylococcus aureus* are indicated, usually flucloxacillin and amoxicillin, or clarithromycin if there is a history of penicillin allergy. The area of cellulitis should be outlined with a marking pen to monitor treatment response.

Reproduced with permission from Eron, L. J. (2000). Infections of skin and soft tissue: outcomes of a classification scheme. *Clinical Infectious Diseases* 31, 287 (A432)

Further Reading

CREST. *Guidelines on the Management of Cellulitis in Adults.* 2005. Available from: https://www.rcem.ac.uk/docs/External%20Guidance/10n.%20Guidelines%20on%20the%20management%20of%20cellulitis%20in%20adults%20(CREST,%202005.pdf

Eron LJ, Lipsky BA, Low DE, Nathwani D, Tice AD, Volturo GA, et al. Managing skin and soft tissue infections: expert panel recommendations on key decision points. *Journal of Antimicrobial Chemotherapy.* 2003;52 Supplement 1:i3–i17.

SAQ 6 **Erythroderma**

A 35-year-old male attends the emergency department with a one-day history of a widespread erythematous and scaling skin rash, which is itchy. On further assessment, 90% of his TBS is involved. There is no mucosal involvement. He is haemodynamically stable and apyrexial.

Q1.   What is the likely diagnosis?
Q2.   List four possible causes for this condition.
Q3.   List three potential complications.

Answers

A1.

The likely diagnosis is erythroderma.

A2.

Causes include:

- Atopic dermatitis
- Adverse cutaneous drug reaction
- Psoriasis
- Lymphoma and leukaemia
- Pityriasis rubra pilaris
- Seborrhoeic dermatitis
- Collagen vascular disease
- Vesiculobullous disorders, such as pemphigus and bullous pemphigoid

A3.

Potential complications include:

- Hypothermia
- Peripheral oedema
- Fluid and electrolyte imbalance
- Acute kidney injury
- Heart failure

Erythroderma is rare but needs to be recognized promptly. It is characterized by erythema and scaling covering more than 90% of the body surface area. The most common cause is an exacerbation of chronic skin condition, particularly psoriasis or atopic dermatitis. Certain medications might also trigger erythroderma: carbamazepine, penicillin, and allopurinol. The risks of the widespread erythema include fluid loss, hypothermia, and electrolyte disturbance. Beyond volume support (if needed) and nursing the patient in a warm environment, symptomatic treatment includes antihistamines and steroids (oral or topical). A dermatologist should be involved in the ongoing management.

Further Reading

Okuduwa C, Lambert WC, Schwartz RA, Kubeyinje E, Eitokpah A, Sinha S, et al. Erythroderma: review of a potentially life-threatening dermatosis. *Indian Journal of Dermatology*. 2009;54:1–6.

Chapter 6 **Endocrinology**

SAQ 1 **Thyroid Storm**

A 26-year-old lady presents with a history of intractable nausea, vomiting, and anxiety. She is febrile, tachycardic, and appears agitated and tremulous. She works as a pharmacist and although she will not tell you what she has taken, she admits to taking 'some tablets to help lose weight'

Q1. What is the likely diagnosis?
Q2. What other precipitants may cause this presentation? Give four.
Q3. Which three medications are key to early management?

Answers

A1.

This is likely to be thyroid storm secondary to thyroxine abuse.

A2.

Other precipitants of thyroid storm (often in patients with untreated underlying hyperthyroidism) can include (list four):

- Trauma
- Untreated Graves' disease
- Infection
- Thyroid surgery
- Sudden cessation of medication for hyperthyroidism
- Pregnancy
- Cardiac emergencies
- Certain medications containing iodine amiodarone and iodinated contrast agents (Jod-Basedow phenomenon) and biological agents (α-interferon)
- Pulmonary embolism
- Diabetic ketoacidosis

A3.

Treatment of thyroid storm comprises:

- Non-cardio-specific beta-adrenergic blocking agents to counteract hyperadrenergic effects of thyroid hormone, such as propranolol or esmolol
- Glucocorticoids, such as hydrocortisone, to inhibit conversion of T4 to T3
- Antithyroid medication such as methimazole to reduce thyroid hormone synthesis

The aims of treatment are to reduce synthesis and release of thyroid hormones and to reduce the peripheral actions of circulating thyroid hormone, in addition to treating the precipitating cause.

T3 (triiodothyronine) and T4 (thyroxine) are produced from iodide ions and tyrosine in the follicle cells of the thyroid gland. The rate of production is controlled by thyroid-stimulating hormone (TSH): TSH promotes iodide uptake into the follicle cells. Although most of the enzymes produced are T4, T3 is the main effector of thyroid hormones: among many other functions, it raises the basal metabolic rate (and is therefore often used as drug of abuse for weight loss). T4 gets converted to T3 by different enzymes in the hepatic, renal, and peripheral tissues.

When a patient is thyrotoxic, the excess T3 can lead to tachycardia, confusion, and pyrexia (often mistaken for a septic patient) and conversely psychosis and agitation may be the only signs of hyper-thyroidism (often mistaken as 'that mental health patient').

The chemical approach to management is as follows; the beta-blocker (often propranolol) inhibits the adrenergic stimulus and therefore reduces symptoms. Hydrocortisone reduces the conversion from T4 to T3. Drugs from the thioamide group (e.g. thiamazole) stop the binding of iodide to tyrosine, hence reducing the production of T4 and T3. Propylthiouracil (PTU) works in the same manner to reduce thyroxine production. Later treatment ought to include colestyramine, which can help bind and excrete excess thyroid hormone. The British National Formulary (BNF) recommends starting with IV fluids, IV 5 mg propranolol, and 100 mg hydrocortisone.

Further Reading

Martini F, Ober WC (2004). *Fundamentals of Anatomy and Physiology*, 6th edition. San Francisco, CA: *Pearson Education International*, pp. 619–26.
McMillen B, Dhillon MS, Yong-Yow S. A rare case of thyroid storm. *BMJ Case Reports*. 2016; 10.1136/bcr-2016-214603.

SAQ 2 **Hyperglycaemic Hyperosmolar State**

A 75-year-old male is brought to hospital in a confused state. He is severely dehydrated. His venous blood glucose is 50 mmol/L

Q1. List three diagnostic criteria for the hyperglycaemic hyperosmolar state.
Q2. In what ways would management differ from that of diabetic ketoacidosis?
Q3. How do you calculate plasma osmolality?

Answers

A1.

The diagnosis of hyperglycaemic hyperosmolar state requires (three from):

- Severe hyperglycaemia (> 30 mmol/L)
- Hyperosmolarity (>320 mosmol/kg)
- Severe volume depletion with prerenal uraemia
- Absence of acidosis (pH >7.3 or HCO_3> 15 mmol/L)
- Minimal or absent ketonaemia (<3 mmol/L)

A2.

The specific issues associated with treatment of the hyperglycaemic hyperosmolar state include:

- Do not start an insulin infusion initially.
- Only start insulin fixed infusion (rate 0.05 units/hr) once glucose stops falling with IV fluids (0.9% saline).
- If the osmolality is not improving despite fluids AND glucose is not reducing, consider 0.45% sodium chloride.

A3.

Plasma osmolality = 2 × sodium + urea + glucose (in mmol/L).

The hyperosmolar hyperglycaemic state (HHS) is dangerous: it has a higher mortality than diabetic ketoacidosis (DKA) and requires rapid recognition and aggressive management. The clinical presentation is more insidious and therefore enough time passes for significant metabolic derangements to occur. It is estimated that by the time of diagnosis with HHS, the patient is water depleted by about 100–200 ml/kg. Aim to achieve a positive fluid balance of 3–6 litres by 12 hours of treatment. The aggressive fluid resuscitation will reduce blood glucose levels: aim for a drop in blood glucose of 5 mmol/L/hr. Some element of ketosis can occur in HHS and therefore the defining criteria allow up to 3 mmol/L of ketonaemia. A significant acidosis (pH <7.30) can occur in a mixed picture of

HHS and DKA. The management needs to be adapted accordingly in those cases. Patients with HHS are at high risk of thrombotic events: MI, CVA, DVTs. Therefore, all patients admitted will require thromboprophylaxis if not contraindicated.

Further Reading

JBDS. *Management of the Hyperosmolar Hyperglycaemic State (HHS) in Adults with Diabetes.* 2012. Joint British Diabetes Societies Inpatient Care Group. Available from: https://diabetes-resources-production.s3-eu-west-1.amazonaws.com/diabetes-storage/migration/pdf/JBDS-IP-HHS-Adults.pdf

SAQ 3 **Tired and Unwell**

A young man presents to your emergency department. He has recently been treated for a flare up of inflammatory bowel disease (IBD). He reports feeling tired and unwell with abdominal pain, muscle cramps, nausea, and vomiting. He says this feels very different to his IBD flares. His blood tests show him to have a slightly low blood glucose, a moderately low sodium, and a slightly raised potassium and creatinine.

Q1. What diagnosis should you suspect?
Q2. What other precipitants are there of this diagnosis? Give four.
Q3. What should your treatment be?

Answers

A1.

An Addisonian crisis in a patient likely to have recently stopped a course of steroid therapy. Adrenal insufficiency could be acutely caused by:

- Septic shock with the precipitant causing adrenal haemorrhage (Waterhouse–Friderichsen syndrome)
- Pituitary tumour or surgery
- Adrenal surgery

A2.

Other precipitants (in those with underlying, unknown, or undertreated adrenal insufficiency) may include (list four):

- Infections
- Injury
- Surgery
- Burns
- Pregnancy
- Anaesthesia
- Cardiac insult
- Allergic reactions
- Hypoglycaemic attacks in diabetics

A3.

Treatment should include hydration with normal saline and intravenous hydrocortisone (100–200 mg intravenous bolus).

Mineralocorticoid replacement is only required if the cause is found or known to be primary adrenal insufficiency. In the first instance (and particularly in the emergency department), hydrocortisone exerts adequate mineralocorticoid activity. Of note, it is possible to develop an Addisonian crisis even while on replacement steroids as requirements can surge in situations of stress (infection, infarction, and so on). The hypotension often improves with administration of hydrocortisone.

Further Reading

Charmandari E, Nicolaides NC, Chrousos GP. Adrenal insufficiency. *Lancet*. 2014;383(9935):2152–67.

SAQ 4 **Blue Feet**

You see a 65-year-old male with poorly controlled diabetes mellitus, whose legs appear as in Fig. 6.1.

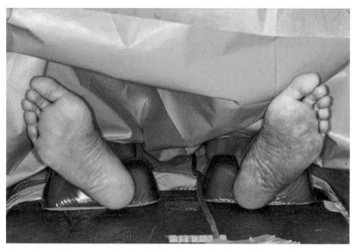

Fig. 6.1 Reproduced from Thompson, M. et al. (2016). *Oxford Textbook of Vascular Surgery*. Oxford University Press. © Oxford University Press 2016. Reproduced with permission of the licensor via PLSClear.

Q1. What diagnosis are you concerned about in Fig. 6.1?
Q2. What classic features of this would you be seeking?
Q3. Other than analgesia, oxygen, and fluids, what key treatment should usually be started without delay?

Answers

A1.

The diagnosis to be concerned about is acute limb ischaemia.

A2.

The six Ps of acute ischaemia include pain, pallor, paraesthesia, paralysis, perishingly cold, and pulselessness.

A3.

Specific initial management involves administration of 5000 units of unfractionated heparin to prevent clot propagation, however an infusion needs starting if intervention will be delayed.

The six Ps are:

Pain: Rest pain is common (worst distally) although the history may be of intermittent claudication prior to the acute presentation. Hanging the legs over the side of the bed may improve perfusion and therefore pain. If passive movement worsens pain, this may indicate developing compartment syndrome.

Pallor: The classic acute appearance is of a white limb although those with chronic ischaemia may have a very pink foot due to long-standing compensation via vasodilatation. Buerger's test may, in chronic ischaemia, demonstrate pallor on elevation and then erythema on dependency.

Paraesthesia: More than half of acute limb ischaemia cases will demonstrate numbness as sensory nerves are smaller than their motor counterparts and so will be preferentially affected.

Paralysis: If this is present it suggests poor prognosis due to the indication of irreversible ischaemia.

Perishingly cold: This should be tested for using the back of the examiner's hand and compared to the other limb.

Pulselessness: Although this is an essential feature to check for, it is very unreliable clinically; therefore, arterial Doppler is needed to measure Ankle Brachial Pressure Index.

Once identified, options for treatment include thrombolysis (either pharmacological or mechanical) or revascularization. This will depend on your local availability of vascular expertise and urgency.

Further Reading

Darwood R. *RCEM—Acute Limb Ischaemia*. 2013. Available from: http://www.rcemlearning.co.uk/references/acute-limb-ischaemia/

SAQ 5 **Diabetic Ketoacidosis (DKA)**

A 24-year-old man is brought into the resuscitation room with a low Glasgow Coma Score. Your Foundation Year 2 trainee has just assessed him and thinks this is a clear case of diabetic ketoacidosis (DKA). To make this case educational, you ask him a few questions:

Q1. What are the biochemical criteria for diagnosing DKA?
Q2. What treatment would you start?
Q3. What should be done if glucose falls below 14 mmol/L?

Answers

A1.

The biochemical criteria for diagnosing DKA include:

- pH <7.30
- HCO3 <15
- Glucose >11
- Ketonuria >2 or ketonaemia >3 mmol/L

A2.

Fluid resuscitation should be commenced immediately. If the patient is not shocked, start with 1 litre 0.9% sodium chloride over the first hour, followed by 1 litre over the subsequent two hours, twice. Start a fixed rate insulin infusion at a rate of 0.1 unit/kg (50 units of human soluble insulin—Actrapid or Humulin S—is made up to 50 ml with 0.9% sodium chloride solution)

A3.

If glucose falls below 14 mmol/L, continue the 0.9% sodium chloride infusion, but run concurrently a 10% glucose infusion at 125 ml/hour.

The joint British Diabetes Society document is a crucial document for every emergency department trainee to be familiar with. The answers given here highlight the key components but other points of note are: no need for insulin bolus on initiation of insulin infusion; continue the patient's long-acting insulin injections even while on the fixed insulin infusion; do not use colloids in the presence of shock.

With the introduction of SGLT-2 inhibitors to control glucose, more cases of euglycaemic ketoacidosis have been noted: whenever you have a patient with severe acidosis and normal glucose, check their regular medications.

Further Reading

JBDS. 2013. *The Management of Diabetic Ketoacidosis in Adults.* Joint British Diabetes Societies Inpatient Care Group. Available from: https://www.diabetes.org.uk/resources-s3/2017-09/Management-of-DKA-241013.pdf

SAQ 6 **Hypoglycaemia**

A 74-year-old diabetic male presents to your emergency department with an acute deterioration of his cognitive function. You suspect he may be hypoglycaemic.

Q1. Define hypoglycaemia.
Q2. List three neurological symptoms you may find.
Q3. List three non-iatrogenic causes of hypoglycaemia.

Answers

A1.

Hypoglycaemia is defined as a blood glucose level less than 3 mmol/L (some sources quote 4 mmol/L).

A2.

Neurological symptoms of hypoglycaemia include (list three):

- Odd behaviour
- Drowsiness
- Confusion
- Seizure
- Speech difficulty
- Irritability
- Incoordination

A3.

Spontaneous hypoglycaemia can be due to (list three):

- Addison's disease
- Pituitary insufficiency
- Liver failure
- Malaria
- Insulinomas
- Extrapancreatic tumours

Hypoglycaemia can mimic many pathologies and it is one of the first bedside tests emergency physicians tend to perform with an acutely deteriorating patient (whether it be due to fear of the embarrassment of missing something 'simple' or because we can easily 'fix it'). If the patient is conscious, oral glucose is a great solution (note: Lucozade drinks often used to be prescribed due to their high sugar content; as of 2017, the contents have reduced from 17 g/100 ml to 8.9 g/100 ml); 1 mg glucagon subcutaneous, intramuscular, or intravenous can be useful, but will fail to improve the blood sugar if the patient has low glycogen stores (liver failure, chronic alcoholic) or is on sulphonylurea medication. Different concentrations of glucose exist: the textbook answer of 50 ml of 50% can still be used. It is tricky to infuse (sticky) and can damage vessels. If there are no concerns about overloading the patient, 250 ml of 10% glucose contains as much glucose as 50 ml of 50% (i.e. 25 g). If you need to give 50% glucose, try to use a large vein and flush it with normal saline after administration).

Further Reading

JBDS. *The Hospital Management of Hypoglycaemia in Adults with Diabetes Mellitus. Joint British Diabetic Societies-Inpatient Care Group (JBDS-IP) Guidelines.* Revised September 2013. Available from: http://www.diabetologists-abcd.org.uk/JBDS/JBDS_HypoGuideline_FINAL_280218.pdf

Chapter 7 **ENT Surgery**

SAQ 1 **Sore Throat**

A 21-year-old university student comes into the department complaining of a sore throat. The triage nurse, who seems unconvinced, tells you she should probably have gone to her general practitioner but said she couldn't get an appointment. You mindfully hold back judgement and decide at the very least you will be able to do some health education with this lady.

Q1. Running through some important differential diagnoses in your mind, what features would make you question if this was a peritonsillar abscess? List at least five.
Q2. Considering this lady's age and risk factors, what triad might suggest infectious mononucleosis?
Q3. If this was a viral or bacterial streptococcal infection how long are her symptoms likely to last?

Answers

A1.

Features of peritonsillar abscess include (five from):

- Severe pain in the pharynx
- Dysphagia
- Drooling
- Trismus
- Speech altered as if a 'hot potato' is in her mouth
- Swollen peritonsillar area
- Medial displacement of tonsil
- Uvula moved contralaterally
- Swollen and erythematous soft palate

Peritonsillar abscess can be life threatening due to the possibility of:

- airway compromise
- aspiration of the contents of the abscess
- vascular involvement.

A2.

Infectious mononucleosis is suggested by a triad of:

- Sore throat
- Fever
- Lymphadenopathy

The pain of the sore throat is worst over 3–5 days then settles over 7–10 days. The patient feels generally unwell disproportionate to the clinical picture. The fever usually reaches 38–39°C, cervical nodes are symmetrically enlarged (most often posterior cervical but commonly submandibular and anterior cervical) and mildly tender. There is usually tonsillar enlargement. A red and exudative palate is possible, alongside palatal petechiae. Bradycardia is usual, and about half have splenomegaly. Less commonly you may find jaundice, hepatomegaly, or a rash.

A3.

40% resolve in 3 days, 85% resolve in 1 week regardless whether it is streptococcal or viral.

The Centor score has been developed to predict Group A Beta-haemolytic Streptococcus infection: if the Centor score is 3–4, the patient is at increased risk of bacterial infection and consequently would benefit from oral antibiotics. The four Centor criteria are:

- Absence of cough
- History of fever
- Presence of tonsillar exudate
- Presence of tender cervical lymphadenopathy

Data from Centor, R.M. et al. The diagnosis of strep throat in adults in the emergency room. *Medical Decision Making.* 1 (3): 239–246. doi:10.1177/0272989x8100100304. PMID 6763125.

If no Centor criteria are present, antibiotics are not recommended.

A more recent scoring system developed is the FeverPAIN score to predict the likelihood of isolating Streptococcus on a throat swab.

Further Reading

Little P, Hobbs FD, Moore M, Mant D, Williamson I, McNulty C, et al. Clinical score and rapid antigen detection test to guide antibiotic use for sore throats: randomised controlled trial of PRISM (primary care streptococcal management) *British Medical Journal.* 2013;347:f5806.

NICE. *Sore Throat—Acute—CKS.* 2015. Available from: http://cks.nice.org.uk/sore-throat-acute#!scenario

SAQ 2 **Epistaxis I**

An 85-year-old male is brought to the emergency department with persistent epistaxis. He is noted to be hypertensive (blood pressure 200/110 mm Hg), and on an oral anticoagulant (rivaroxaban).

Q1. What initial measures would be required to stop the bleeding?
Q2. What features indicate posterior epistaxis?
Q3. There is no ENT surgeon on site, and the patient continues to bleed. What treatment options are available to facilitate safe transfer to another hospital?

Answers

A1.

Local haemostatic measures, such as local pressure (patient presses firmly on alae) or nasal packing, should be initiated.

Cotton swabs soaked with a lidocaine/adrenaline mix can lead to vasoconstriction and analgesia when time comes to cauterize an anterior bleed. Packing the nasal cavity can be distressing, so consider the use of anxiolytics (any benzodiazepine intravenous). RAPID RHINO nasal pack needs to be soaked in sterile water, NOT saline. There is no reversal agent for rivaroxaban (factor Xa inhibitor) currently available. You can consider prothrombin complex concentrate after discussion with a haematologist for life threatening bleeding.

A2.

Features indicating posterior epistaxis include:

- Older age
- Bilateral epistaxis
- Large volume of blood in oropharynx
- Persistent bleeding in the presence of adequate anterior nasal packing

A3.

Prior to safe transfer, the following interventions can be attempted to control bleeding

- Nasal sponges or tampons, for example, Merocel®; Rapid Rhino® (carboxymethylcellulose-infused fabric)
- Balloon devices (e.g. Brighton balloon; these are triple-lumen double balloon devices)
- Foley catheter (size 10, 12, or 14)—this is an unlicensed use; the balloon is inflated in the postnasal space

Although high blood pressure is noted to be reasonably common in patients with nosebleeds, studies have been unable to find a convincing causative relationship because of confounders such as stress of the episode or white coat hypertension.

When the patient presents for the first time, there is usually no need to investigate using blood tests unless there is a specific concern. If large blood loss is suspected due to recurrent or heavy bleeding or anaemia is questioned, then a full blood count is appropriate. If there is suspicion of a clotting disorder or anticoagulation dose may need adjusting, then it is appropriate to do coagulation studies.

Epistaxis in the following patients should be considered as a trigger for referral:

- Age younger than 2 years as this is often associated with significant trauma or a serious underlying issue
- Symptoms suggestive of neoplasm, including facial pain, nasal obstruction, rhinorrhoea, or cranial nerve lesions (such as double vision or facial numbness)
- Patients with an underlying known cause are likely to need to see a specialist
- Any patient who has required nasal packing
- Any patient who remains haemodynamically compromised with epistaxis as the cause
- The acuity of the referral is dependent of local policies and availability of outpatient consultation

Further Reading

BMJ. *Best Practice: Epistaxis*. 2016. Available from: https://bestpractice.bmj.com/best-practice/monograph/421/step-by-step.html

NICE. *Epistaxis (Nosebleeds)—NICE CKS*. 2015. Available from: http://cks.nice.org.uk/epistaxis-nosebleeds

SAQ 3 **Vertigo**

Your Foundation Year 2 (FY2) trainee has seen a 75-year-old male, who presents with the acute onset of 'dizziness' and is unable to walk due to ataxia. He wants to refer the patient to the stroke unit.

Q1.   What features make central vertigo more likely in this situation?
Q2.   List two features suggestive of benign paroxysmal positional vertigo.
Q3.   What emergency department treatments are available for the management of peripheral vertigo?

Answers

A1.

Central vertigo is more likely with the following:

- Constant vertigo
- Not positional or related to movement
- Nausea and vomiting are infrequent
- No hearing loss or tinnitus
- Concomitant cerebellar or brain stem signs or symptoms: diplopia, dysphagia, dysarthria, facial weakness or numbness, ataxia, hemiparesis
- Nystagmus not inhibited by ocular fixation
- Non-fatigable, multidirectional nystagmus
- Cerebrovascular risk factors

A2.

Features of benign paroxysmal positional vertigo include (two from):

- Typically presents with acute onset of severe dizziness
- Each episode is brief (usually 10–20 seconds but may last as long as 90 seconds) rather than persistent, the episodes occurring in clusters
- Vertigo is precipitated by positional changes of the head

A3.

Peripheral vertigo can be treated with:

- Vestibular sedatives, which include antihistamines, anticholinergic agents, and benzodiazepines
- BPPV can be treated with a canalith repositioning procedure which moves the canaliths from the posterior semicircular canal back to the saccule (Semont or Epley's manoeuvres)

A concern for every emergency department doctor is to be able to differentiate between a 'central or peripheral cause' for the patient presenting with vertigo. A validated examination sequence is the HINTS test: Head Impulse, Nystagmus, and Test of Skew. The head impulse tests for the vestibulo-ocular reflex (VOR): when a central lesion is present, the VOR reflex is intact. Nystagmus due to peripheral pathology tends to be horizontal and unidirectional. Vertical nystagmus could indicate a central lesion. The Test of Skew is due to a vertical ocular misalignment secondary to a central cause. The link to an excellent YouTube video is linked in the following list of further reading recommendations.

Further Reading

BMJ Best Practice. *Vertigo*. 2017. Available from: http://bestpractice.bmj.com/best-practice/monograph/965.html

Johns P. *A Basic, Simplified Approach to the Dizzy Patient Part 1* [Video]. Available from: https://www.youtube.com/watch?v=9fQInDLVeCE&app=desktop

Kattah JC, Talkad AV, Wang DZ, Hsieh Y-H, Newman-Toker DE. H.I.N.T.S. to diagnose stroke in the acute vestibular syndrome—three-step bedside oculomotor exam more sensitive than early MRI diffusion-weighted imaging. *Stroke*. 2009;40(11):3504–10.

SAQ 4 **Peritonsillar Abscess**

A 26-year-old male has been referred to the emergency department with sore throat and a general practitioner's note reading 'please see, has? quinsy'

Q1. List five clinical features indicating quinsy.
Q2. List three treatment options.
Q3. List two complications.

Answers

A1.

Clinical features suggesting quinsy include:

- Severe sore throat, with or without referred ear pain
- A muffled 'hot potato' voice
- Trismus
- Halitosis
- Dysphagia, with drooling of saliva
- Unilateral tonsillar swelling with displacement of the uvula
- Cervical lymphadenopathy

A2.

Treatment options include:

- Intravenous antibiotic therapy
- Needle aspiration
- Incision and drainage of the abscess
- Emergency tonsillectomy

A3.

Potential complications of quinsy include:

- Extension into contiguous deep neck spaces (e.g. parapharyngeal abscess)
- Airway obstruction
- Suppurative thrombophlebitis of the internal jugular vein (Lemierre's disease)
- Mediastinitis
- Aspiration pneumonia and lung abscess
- Erosion of carotid artery with massive haemorrhage

Quinsy is most commonly due to *Streptococcus pyogenes* and *Staphylococcus aureus*. Smoking is a risk factor. Recent studies indicate the use of ultrasound in differentiating a peritonsillar abscess and peritonsillar cellulitis. If further imaging is required, a computed tomography (CT) scan with contrast is the preferred method (note an estimated dose of 3 mSv). CT can provide further details if deep space infection is suspected and will help guide management.

Further Reading

Galioto NJ. Peritonsillar abscess. *American Family Physician*. 2008;77:199–202.

Secko M, Sivitz A. Think ultrasound first for peritonsillar swelling. *American Journal of Emergency Medicine*. 2015;33(4):569–72.

SAQ 5 **Nasal Fracture**

A 32-year-old male has been punched in the face during a fight and attends the emergency department with a painful deformed nose. You suspect a nasal fracture

Q1. What associated complicating injuries should you look for (list three)?
Q2. What treatments may be necessary (list two)?
Q3. When is imaging indicated?

Answers

A1.

It is important to exclude:

- Septal haematoma (subperichondrial bleeding); failure to treat may lead to septal cartilage necrosis with a saddle-nose deformity
- Septal dislocation
- Nasoethmoidal fracture (flattening of the nasal bridge; periorbital bruising; traumatic telecanthus; cerebrospinal fluid leak)
- Cerebrospinal fluid (CSF) leakage, associated with fracture of the cribriform plate of the ethmoid

A2.

Possible treatment for a nasal fracture may include:

- Incision and drainage of septal haematoma
- Early closed reduction

A3.

CT scanning is indicated if there is a suspected basal skull fracture with cerebrospinal fluid leak, or with suspected nasoethmoidal fracture.

A septal haematoma can lead to ischaemic necrosis of the septum: prompt drainage is often recommended (but rarely performed in the ED). Drainage involves piercing the haematoma with a small scalpel blade and evacuating the clot: it is important to pack the nasal cavity bilaterally to reduce the risk of reaccumulation. Septal dislocation can lead to difficulty in breathing through one nostril, cosmetic and psychological side effects, and even sleep apnoea. An ENT surgeon can attempt to relocate it in due course (as with fractures, they should be followed up within 14 days at the very latest).

Further Reading

Kucik CJ. Management of acute nasal fractures. *American Family Physician*. 2004;70: 1315–20.

SAQ 6 **Otitis Externa**

A 65-year-old male with type 2 diabetes mellitus attends the emergency department with acute pain and swelling in the right pinna, which developed two days ago and is progressively worsening. There is no history of trauma.

Q1. List four clinical features of acute otitis externa.
Q2. List three factors which can predispose to this condition.
Q3. How would you initiate management in the emergency department? List three interventions.

Answers

A1.

The features of acute otitis externa include:

- Itching, pain, swelling, and redness involving the external auditory meatus and canal
- Serous or purulent discharge, with crusting of the skin of the canal
- Conductive hearing loss
- Pain on chewing food
- Tenderness of the tragus
- Pain on manipulation of the pinna
- Pre- and postauricular and anterior cervical adenopathy

A2.

Predisposing factors include warm and humid environment, anatomical narrowing of the external auditory canal with wax impaction, trauma from the use of cotton buds or other material to clean the ear canal, use of hearing aids, and swimming, especially in polluted water.

A3.

- Obtain a wound swab for culture and sensitivity
- Commence a course of antibiotic/steroid drops to provide cover against *Pseudomonas* and *Staphylococcus*
- Oral antibiotics can be considered with spread of cellulitis to the face, systemic signs of infection, or in immunosuppressed states
- Ensure follow-up, so that suction clearance of debris and purulent discharge in the outer ear canal under microscopic control can be performed if there is poor response to medical treatment

Ibuprofen and paracetamol are often sufficient analgesia, NICE recommends codeine in severe pain. There is no evidence of benefit of topical antibiotics with steroids when compared to antibiotics without steroids. Do not use aminoglycosides if the tympanic membrane is perforated. If perforation is suspected/confirmed, consider quinolone containing drops. In mild cases, use acetic acid drops.

Further Reading

CKS. *Otitis Externa*. 2018. Available from: https://cks.nice.org.uk/otitis-externa#!scenario:1

Rosenfeld RM, Schwartz SR, Cannon CR, Roland PS, Simon GR, Kumar KA, et al. Clinical practice guideline: acute otitis externa. *Otolaryngology: Head and Neck Surgery*. 2014;150 (1 Supplement):s1–s24.

SAQ 7 **Nasal Foreign Bodies**

Children are inquisitive and may introduce foreign objects through their nostrils, often unwitnessed.

Q1. List three clinical features suggestive of a retained nasal foreign body.
Q2. What techniques can be considered for foreign body removal in children?
Q3. List four complications of nasal foreign bodies.

Answers

A1.

A retained nasal foreign body should be suspected in the presence of:

- Unilateral foul smelling, mucopurulent, often blood-stained, nasal discharge
- Unilateral vestibulitis with nasal excoriation
- Persistent unilateral epistaxis
- Foul odour originating from the body (bromhidrosis) or mouth (halitosis)

A2.

Methods for removal of nasal foreign bodies in children include:

- Positive pressure technique, using the 'magic kiss'—ask the parent to block the contralateral unaffected nostril and blow gently into the mouth, leading to positive pressure through mouth
- Instrumentation: bayonet or alligator forceps; flange-tipped suction catheter; right-angled hook; balloon catheter; Katz extractor (balloon catheter device)
- Removal under general anaesthesia, with pharyngeal pack

A3.

Complications associated with nasal foreign body retention include:

- Sinusitis
- Nasal septal perforation (especially with button batteries and magnets)
- Orbital cellulitis
- Aspiration with acute airway obstruction
- Rhinoliths

Foreign objects in ears or noses tend to occur more frequently in children under the age of 10 years. In the younger children, the nostril seems to be the preferred orifice for insertion. While the 'magic kiss' or 'mother's kiss' can be successful, one has to be ready to extract objects using other tools: crocodile forceps are very useful but it is important to remember that in children, the best attempt is the first one: cooperation dwindles rapidly in a four-year-old. To increase your chances of success, the use of topical anaesthetic should be considered. Lidocaine does kill insects trapped in ear canals, so apply this first prior to attempting to remove the moth from an ear.

Further Reading

Davies PH, Benger JR. Foreign bodies in the nose and ear: a review of techniques for removal in the emergency department. *Emergency Medicine Journal* 2000; 17:91–4.

Kalan A, Tariq M. Foreign bodies in the nasal cavities: a comprehensive review of the aetiology, diagnostic pointers, and therapeutic measures. *Postgraduate Medical Journal*. 2000;76:484–7.

Kiger JR, Brenkert TE, Losek JD. Nasal foreign body removal in children. *Paediatric Emergency Care*. 2008;24:785–92.

Chapter 8 Environmental Medicine and Toxicology

SAQ 1 **Serotonin Syndrome**

At 2:11 am you receive a pre-alert for a priority call: a 19-year-old man has been out clubbing with his friends. After taking MDMA (3,4-methylenedioxymethamphetamine), he was found to be agitated, requiring restraint.

Q1. You wonder whether he might be developing signs/symptoms of serotonin syndrome. Give two features of serotonin syndrome (other than agitation and hypertension).

Q2. On arrival, he is agitated and hypertensive. What first-line medication would you give to address the blood pressure?

Q3. Name two prescription medications that could give rise to similar presentation.

Answers

A1.

Tachycardia and hyperthermia are significant features.

Serotonin syndrome is a potentially life-threatening syndrome characterized by a triad of autonomic instability, neuromuscular hyperactivity, and alteration of mental status. A list of possible answers follows:

Central nervous system:
  Agitation
  Confused
  Decreased level of consciousness
  Seizure

Motor:
  Hyperreflexia
  Myoclonus
  Rigidity
  Incoordination
  Tremor

Autonomic:
  Sweating
  Diarrhoea
  Fever
  Hypertension
  Tachycardia
  Mydriasis

A2.

Diazepam. The agitation is best treated with intravenous boluses of benzodiazepine (e.g. 0.1–0.3 mg/kg diazepam). This in itself will often have an effect on the blood pressure. If this fails, a glyceryl trinitrate infusion can be used, starting at a rate of 1–2 mg/hour, and adjusting as needed.

A3.

Serotonergic drugs include selective serotonin reuptake inhibitors and monoamine oxidase inhibitors. The modes of action include inhibition of serotonin uptake or metabolism, increase of serotonin synthesis or release, or activation of serotonin receptors.

The list of potential culprits unfortunately is long and the following are correct answers:

Selective serotonin reuptake inhibitors (SSRI)
Monoamine oxidase inhibitors (MAOI)
Serotonin-norepinephrine reuptake inhibitors
Tricyclic antidepressants
5-HT$_3$ antagonists
Opiates, including tramadol
Triptans

Further Reading

RCEM Learning. *Drug Induced Hyperthermia*. 2018. Available from: https://www.rcemlearning.co.uk/references/drug-induced-hyperthermia/

SAQ 2 **Chemical Incident**

Five males are sent to your emergency department having been exposed to a white powdered chemical at their workplace, which may be potentially toxic. A supervisor is bringing an information sheet describing the nature of this chemical.

Q1. List a source of information that can be contacted for guidance to help manage this incident.
Q2. What technique can be used for decontamination following non-caustic chemical exposures?
Q3. How would you decontaminate victims of caustic chemical exposure?

Answers

A1.

Sources of information include TOXBASE, which is the online clinical toxicology database of the National Poisons Information Service (NPIS) (https://www.toxbase.org), which requires password access.

Other answers could be:

Clinical biochemist/toxicologist in the hospital

UK National Poisons Information Service (0344 892011)

A2.

The most important technique is to use a dry material to blot rather than brush off the chemical.

A normal process would be: prompt disrobing to underwear within 15–20 minutes of exposure, followed by dry decontamination using dry absorbent materials such as cloths, paper hand towels (blue roll), incontinence pads, or wound dressings, to blot rather than rub exposed skin surfaces. As a final stage, any long or thick matted hair should be washed in running water, with the person leaning forwards. Double bag all waste material arising from disrobing and decontamination in clinical waste bags (or equivalent) and tie for disposal at a later stage. Follow local procedures for rerobing, handling of personal items, and hazardous waste management (should be within each department's major incident protocol).

A3.

Wet decontamination with water for 45–90 seconds, ideally with a washing aid such as a cloth.
Water can be used from any available source: taps; showers; hose-reels or sprinklers.
Double bag in clinical waste bags (or equivalent), tied for disposal at a later stage.

Further Reading

TOXBASE. Available from: https://www.toxbase.org [Online database requiring preregistration].

SAQ 3 Major Incident

You are working in the emergency department when a major incident has been declared.

Q1. List two personnel or agencies that can declare a major incident.
Q2. What are the three levels of command in the command and control structure for major incident management?
Q3. List two patterns in which a major incident could arise.

Answers

A1.

A major incident can be declared by:

- Ambulance service
- Fire brigade

Other suitable answers are:

- Police service
- Nurse in charge or consultant in emergency department or silver/gold command of hospital

A2.

The levels of command are:

- Gold: strategic
- Silver: tactical
- Bronze: operational

A3.

The different ways a major incident can develop are:

- Big bang: a serious transport accident, explosion, or series of smaller incidents
- Rising tide: developing infectious disease epidemic, capacity/staffing crisis, overseas incident
- Cloud on the horizon: major chemical or nuclear release developing elsewhere and needing preparatory action, dangerous epidemics, armed conflict
- Headline news: wave of public or media alarm over health issue or perceived threat
- CBRN release: deliberate or accidental release of chemical, biological, radiological, nuclear, or explosive materials
- Business continuity
- Mass casualties
- Preplanned major events: sports fixtures, mass gatherings, demonstrations, air shows, race meetings

Further Reading

Blom L, Black JJM. Major incidents. *British Medical Journal.* 2014;348:g1144.

SAQ 4 **Carbon Monoxide Poisoning**

A 35-year-old woman has been rescued from a house fire. She is being managed in the resuscitation room. Your FY2 trainee has never seen a case with suspected carbon monoxide poisoning and would like to know more.

Q1. What are the signs and symptoms of carbon monoxide poisoning?
Q2. What first treatment is required for carbon monoxide poisoning?
Q3. What are the criteria for transfer to a hyperbaric chamber?

Answers

A1.

The most common first symptom is a headache. Other symptoms are nausea and vomiting, dizziness or vertigo, shortness of breath, and altered consciousness. The symptoms are non-specific and mimic viral infections, flu, and food poisoning. Symptoms may occur in other household members, including pets. When taking a history for a patient with headache, remember the possibility of chronic carbon monoxide poisoning. An easy way to remember the questions is to remember 'COMA': are any **C**ohabitants suffering from headaches? Does the headache get better when **O**utside? Are your gas appliances regularly **M**aintained? Do you have a carbon monoxide **A**larm at home?

A2.

The mainstay of treatment is high-flow oxygen. Remember the 1-23-4 rule: on high-flow oxygen the half-life of CO is 1 hour; in a hyperbaric chamber it is 23 minutes; on air it is 4 hours.

A3.

What are the criteria for transfer to a hyperbaric chamber?

Transfer to a hyperbaric chamber should be considered if the patient has been unconscious at any point, has a COHb of more than 20%, has had a seizure, any neurological deficits, or is pregnant. Evidence of myocardial ischaemia is also an indicator for discussion of transfer. NB: COHb up to 8% can be normal in smokers, who also have a higher tolerance for CO.

Further Reading

Department of Health statement. Available from: https://assets.publishing.service.gov.uk/government/uploads/system/uploads/attachment_data/file/260211/Carbon_Monoxide_Letter_2013_FinalforPub.pdf

SAQ 5 **Burns**

A 7-year-old boy attends with a scald to his chest and arms. You estimate the total area of burn to be approximately 10%.

Q1. How much fluid would you give him in the first 8 hours?
Q2. What analgesia would you provide?
Q3. List three features of full-thickness burns.

Answers

A1.

560 ml of crystalloid. The estimated weight for a 7-year-old child is (3× age +7) 28 kg. The Parkland formula estimates the fluid requirement to start resuscitation: 4 × weight (kg) × total burn surface area (%) = amount in millilitres (1120 ml). Half of the total amount is to be given in the first 8 hours, the remaining half over the following 16 hours.

A2.

Analgesia can be provided by intranasal diamorphine 0.1 mg/kg. Administering intranasal 0.1 mg/kg diamorphine in a 0.2 ml volume is an efficient way to manage initial pain. Covering the burns with cling film also helps to relieve pain.

A3.

Full-thickness burns are characterized by (list three):

- A dense white, waxy, charred, or leathery appearance
- Loss of sensation to pinprick
- Absence of blanching on pressure
- Thrombosed vessels within the burnt area
- Eschar (dry black necrotic tissue) formation
- Prolonged time for healing, with severe scarring

Further Reading

British Burns Association. *European Standards: Practice Guidelines for Burn Care*. Available from: http://www.britishburnsassociation.org/european-standards

SAQ 6 **Hypothermia**

A gentleman with no fixed abode is brought in by ambulance. It is snowing outside and he was found in a shop doorway. The paramedics are concerned he is suffering the effects of hypothermia. His body temperature is noted to be 30°C.

Q1. What are the three grades of hypothermia?
Q2. Which electrocardiogram (ECG) finding, though not always present, is pathognomonic of hypothermia?
Q3. Below what temperature should cardioactive drugs be withheld?

Answers

A1

The three grades of hypothermia are:

- Mild: 32–35°C
- Moderate: 28–32°C
- Severe: less than 28°C

A2.

The J-wave (or Osborn wave) is pathognomonic of hypothermia. The J-wave is a deflection just after the QRS complex. Bradycardia is also common, as well as T-wave inversion and prolongation of the QT interval.

A3.

Below 30°C. Below this level, cardioactive drugs can accumulate and reach toxic levels. Warmed IV fluids can help with the general absorption of intravenous medications in the hypothermic patient. At temperatures just above 30°C it is prudent to double intervals between cardioactive drugs if they are to be given. Only give 3 DC shocks if temperature is below 30°C. Continue with DC cardioversion (as per ALS) once core temperature above 30°C.

Further Reading

BMJ. Hypothermia. 2016. Available from: http://bestpractice.bmj.com/best-practice/monograph/654.html
Life in the Fast Lane. *Hypothermia*. Available from: https://lifeinthefastlane.com/ccc/hypothermia/

SAQ 7 **Lightning Injury**

A family of five attends your emergency department, concerned as their house was struck by lightning. Relieved, you see that all of them appear well, although you recall that lightning after-effects are not necessarily obvious straight away.

Q1.   Which tissue does lightning preferentially pass through in the human body?
Q2.   What is the mechanism of sudden death in lightning strike?
Q3.   Should cardiac markers be measured?

Answers

A1.

Lightning preferentially passes through nerves. It will travel through nerve preferentially as all electrical energy travels the path with least resistance and in the body the order of least to most resistance is as follows: nerve < blood < muscle < skin < fat < bone.

A2.

Sudden death is the result of simultaneous cardiac arrest alongside respiratory arrest.

   It is to be noted that cardiac arrest has a quicker recovery time than respiratory arrest because of the prolonged effect on the medullary respiratory centre.

A3.

No. Although cardiac markers may be raised, they have not been shown to have any prognostic significance. ECG changes can be varied and may present up to 72 hours after the event.

Further Reading

Life in the Fast Lane. *Lightning Injury*. Available from: https://lifeinthefastlane.com/ccc/lightning-injury/

SAQ 8 **Anaphylaxis**

A 25-year-old female has been stung by bees while in the garden and presents with a sense of constriction in the throat, widespread urticaria and wheezing, and has a heart rate of 110 beats per minute and a blood pressure of 80/50 mm Hg.

Q1. What immediate pharmacological treatments would you recommend?
Q2. What investigation may help with confirmation of the diagnosis?
Q3. When would you prescribe an Epi-Pen®?

Answers

A1.

The immediate treatment of an anaphylactic reaction comprises:

- 0.5 ml of intramuscular adrenaline (1:1000 solution, i.e. 500 mcg)
- Intravenous or intramuscular hydrocortisone 200 mg
- Intravenous or intramuscular chlorphenamine 10 mg

A2.

Serum tryptase levels. Tryptase is an endoprotease exclusively present in mast cells. Normal serum tryptase is less than 12 μg/L. Serum tryptase levels are elevated for 1–6 hours after the event.

Timed blood levels should be taken as soon as possible after emergency treatment and a second sample ideally within 1–2 hours later. The patient should be observed for 6–12 hours post-onset of symptoms. The National Institute for Health and Care Excellence (NICE) recommends that all patients should be offered a referral to a specialist allergy clinic and discharged the patient with an adrenaline injector.

A3.

Epi-Pen® (adrenaline autoinjector) should be prescribed following an anaphylactic episode if there is a continuing risk of a reaction to an identified trigger which cannot be avoided (e.g. peanut allergy, stinging, or biting insect allergy, as part of a comprehensive management plan). It is usually not required following drug-induced anaphylaxis, unless avoidance of exposure is difficult. The Epi-Pen is designed for early treatment of severe reactions in the community.

Further information is available at https://www.rcemlearning.co.uk/references/anaphylaxis/

Further Reading

NICE. *Anaphylaxis: Assessment and Referral After Emergency Treatment CG134*. Available from: https://www.nice.org.uk/guidance/cg134

SAQ 9 **Paracetamol Overdose**

A 28-year-old female has ingested 20 tablets of paracetamol two hours prior to arrival in hospital, along with two glasses of wine.

Q1. What is the initial management for paracetamol poisoning for this person?
Q2. By what mechanism does paracetamol overdose cause toxicity?
Q3. What is the recommended first-line antidote?

Answers

A1.

Check paracetamol levels at 4 hours post-ingestion.

If paracetamol level is above the treatment line, administer a full course of antidote: 21 hours, in three sequential infusion**s**, each containing a different dose of antidote, and based on body weight of the patient: 150 mg/kg in 200 ml 5% glucose over 1 hour followed by 50 mg/kg in 500 ml 5% dextrose over next 4 hours, followed by 100 mg/kg in 1000 ml 5% dextrose over next 16 hours.

A2.

Paracetamol is converted to NAPQI (N-acetyl-p-benzoquinone imine), which is hepatotoxic.

The major products of metabolism of paracetamol in the liver are inactive and non-toxic glucuronide and sulphate conjugates. Most of the drug is metabolized into non-toxic metabolites, but 5–10% is converted by the cytochrome P450 system into the reactive toxic intermediate N-acetyl-p-benzoquinone imine (NAPQI), which is hepatotoxic and nephrotoxic. NAPQI is usually bound to glutathione when paracetamol is taken within therapeutic levels. When excess levels of NAPQI are present, glutathione stores get depleted and hepatotoxicity occurs. Acetylcysteine helps restore glutathione and hence offer protective benefit.

A3.

Acertylcysteine. Methionine is the second-line antidote.

Further Reading

BMJ Best Practice. Available from: http://bestpractice.bmj.com/best-practice/monograph/337/treatment/step-by-step.html
Toxbase. *Paracetemol.* Available from: https://www.toxbase.org/Poisons-Index-A-Z/P-Products/Paracetamol-----------/

SAQ 10 **Methanol Toxicity**

A 66-year-old lady is brought to the resuscitation room with abdominal pain, loose stools, and hypothermia and tachycardia. Her past medical history includes type 2 diabetes mellitus and bipolar disease.

Her venous blood gas on arrival is: pH 6.71, pCO_2 3.69, pO_2 10.4, HCO_3 3.3, BE −31, Na 136, K 5.81, Cl 102, glucose 8.6, lactate 16.57.

Q1. What does the venous gas demonstrate?
Q2. Give three possible differential diagnoses.
Q3. Within 40 minutes of being in the department, she suddenly states she is unable to see. What toxidrome should you consider?

Answers

A1.

A severe metabolic acidosis with respiratory compensation. A dramatic rise in lactate always raises the suspicion of ischaemic tissue, and particularly ischaemic bowel when presentation includes abdominal pain.

A2.

Differential diagnoses include:

* Sepsis
* Ischaemic bowel
* Euglycaemic ketoacidosis

A3.

Methanol overdose.

Note: early visual symptoms can be photophobia, blurring of vision, or painful eye movements and occur 10–24 hours after ingestion of methanol. This can initially be mistaken for an ethanol overdose: confusion, unsteadiness, nausea. The severe metabolic acidosis on a venous blood gas with a high anion gap nevertheless would point to methanol as causation. Methanol is transformed into formic acid which leads to both acidosis and the ophthalmological injuries. Two antidotes are available: ethanol and fomepizole.

Anion gap = (Sodium + Potassium)—(Chloride + Bicarbonate).
The normal range is 12–16 mmol/L.

Further Reading

Toxbase. *Methanol.* Available from: https://www.toxbase.org/Poisons-Index-A-Z/M-Products/ Methanol---------------/

UpToDate. *Diabetic Ketoacidosis and Hyperosmolar Hyperglycemic State in Adults: Clinical Features, Evaluation, and Diagnosis.* Available from: https://www.uptodate.com/contents/diabetic-ketoacidosis-and-hyperosmolar-hyperglycemic-state-in-adults-clinical-features-evaluation-and-diagnosis?source=search_result&search=euglycemic%20dka&selectedTitle=1~150

SAQ 11 **Beta-blocker Overdose**

A 39-year-old lady is brought into your resuscitation room. She is drowsy, with a blood pressure of 105/62 mm Hg and has a pulse rate of 34 bpm. The paramedic found two empty boxes of bisoprolol next to her bed. Your FY2 trainee has given her atropine but this did not have any effect.

Q1. What medication would you suggest him to use next (dose and route).
Q2. Within a few minutes, she arrests, and your team starts the standard advanced life support (ALS) treatment. Beyond ALS treatment, what drug could be used to reduce the toxicity of a beta-blocker overdose?
Q3. If all medical treatment fails, what could be your last option for managing this arrest?

Answers

A1.

Intravenous glucagon 5–10 mg has shown to have some benefit in beta-blocker overdose. High doses of insulin (bolus of 1 unit/kg followed by infusion of 0.5–2 units/kg/hr) and glucose have also been shown to be of benefit.

A2.

A 1.5 ml/kg bolus of 20% Intralipid® followed by an infusion of 0.25–0.5 ml/kg/min over 30–60 minutes, up to 500 ml total.

A3.

Consider VA-ECMO (veno-arterial extracorporeal membrane oxygenation).

Further Reading

Toxbase. *Bisoprolol-Fumarate.* Available from: https://www.toxbase.org/Poisons-Index-A-Z/B-Products/Bisoprolol-Fumarate---/

SAQ 12 **Heat Stroke**

You are working at an aid station at a marathon. A 37-year-old man is brought in after a collapse. Simon is vomiting, confused, has very dry skin, hyperventilating, and hypotensive. He has a core temperature of 41°C.

Q1. What is the likely diagnosis?
Q2. What is the mainstay of treatment for Simon?
Q3. Give two determinants of mortality of this condition?

Answers

A1.

The likely diagnosis is heat stroke.

The differences between heat exhaustion and heat stroke are summarized in Table 8.1.

Table 8.1

Heat exhaustion	Heatstroke
Headache	Neurological dysfunction
Core temperature <40°C	Core temperature >41°C
Vomiting	Dry skin
Malaise	Loss of consciousness
Dizziness	Profuse sweating
Tachycardia	Tachycardia
Orthostatic hypotension	Hyperventilation
Nausea	Seizures
	Vomiting
	Hypotension

A2.

He requires cooling, at a rate of approximately 0.1 degree/minute. Multiple methods for cooling are available. Removing the clothes and spray with fine mist of tepid water, ice packs to groins and axillae, ice water immersion, IV cold saline, and peritoneal lavage are all possible methods of cooling. NB: it is important to control shivering and seizures and monitor urine output.

A3.

Predictors of mortality include duration of elevation of temperature, maximum core temperature, prolonged coma, and acute kidney injury.

Further Reading

RCEM. *2017 Guidelines for Management of Marathon Related Medical Emergencies.* 2017. Available from: http://www.rcem.ac.uk/docs/RCEM%20Guidance/2017%20Guidelines_for_Management_of_Marathon_Related_Medical_Emergencies.pdf

SAQ 13 **Local Anaesthetic Toxicity**

You attend an emergency call in your department. Your ST1 trainee had just finished performing a fascia iliaca block when the patient became unresponsive.

Q1. What are the initial symptoms of lidocaine toxicity?
Q2. What is the treatment for lidocaine toxicity?
Q3. How would you calculate the maximum safe dose of lidocaine?

Answers

A1.

The initial symptoms of lidocaine toxicity are:

- Mouth and tongue numbness or tingling
- Tinnitus
- Confusion followed by seizures and cardiac arrhythmias can occur

A2.

The treatment for lidocaine toxicity is 1.5 ml/kg 20% Intralipid® intravenous bolus over one minute.

Up to three boluses of 1.5 ml/kg at 5-minute intervals if an adequate circulation is not restored, followed by an IV infusion of 20% emulsion at 15 ml/kg/hour, increasing to 30 ml/kg/hour after 5 minutes, if cardiovascular stability not restored. The maximum cumulative dose is 12 ml/kg.

A3.

The maximum safe dose of lidocaine is 3 mg/kg (without adrenaline) or 7 mg/kg (with adrenaline 1: 200 000).

Further Reading

AAGBI. *Management of Severe Local Anaesthetic Toxicity*. 2010. Available from: https://www.aagbi.org/sites/default/files/la_toxicity_2010_0.pdf

SAQ 14 **Anticoagulant Reversal**

A 76-year-old male is brought into your emergency department after a road traffic accident. You note that he is bleeding from an open femoral shaft fracture. He is on warfarin for his atrial fibrillation. His international normalized ratio (INR) is subsequently found to be 5.

Q1. What pharmacological agent would you administer for rapid reversal of his anticoagulant?
Q2. Prior to transfer to the trauma unit, you note that his fibrinogen has fallen below 1.5 g/L. What pharmacological agent should you give to correct this?
Q3. Above what level should you try to keep the platelet count?

Answers

A1.

Prothrombin complex concentrate, which consists of factors II, VII, IX, and X, is recommended for reversal of a supratherapeutic INR in this situation. Four-factor concentrate has superseded three-factor concentrate.

A2.

Cryoprecipitate, which is the precipitate obtained by thawing of fresh frozen plasma, and contains fibrinogen, factor VII, von Willebrand factor, factor XIII, and fibronectin. It is used as a pooled product made up of five single units for the treatment of adults.

A3.

The platelet count should be maintained greater than $75 \times 10^9/L$.

Prothrombin complex concentrate (PCC) is the recommended agent to rapidly reverse warfarin. Four-factor concentrate contains vitamin K-dependent coagulation factors II, VII, IX, X, and vitamin K-dependent coagulation inhibition proteins C and S. The trade names are Beriplex® and Octaplex®. Warfarin-induced anticoagulation can be reversed within ten minutes. Approx. 5 mg intravenous vitamin K should be given with PCC. Cryoprecipitate is created from concentrating fresh frozen plasma and mainly contains factor VIII, von Willebrand factor, and fibrinogen.

Further Reading

RCEM Learning. *Management of the Overanticoagulated Patient*. Available from: https://www.rcemlearning.co.uk/modules/management-of-the-over-anticoagulated-patient/

SAQ 15 **Salicylate Poisoning**

The Psychiatry Liaison Nurse draws your attention to a 25-year-old male who has recently taken an aspirin overdose.

Q1.   Describe the mechanism by which salicylate toxicity causes respiratory alkalosis.
Q2.   Fill in Table 8.2.
Q3.   Describe what is meant by alkalinization of urine.

Table 8.2

	Mg/L	Treatment
Mild		
Moderate		
Severe		

Answers

A1.

This occurs through stimulation of the respiratory centres in the medulla oblongata resulting in tachypnoea and subsequent alkalosis.

A2.

Please see Table 8.3.

Table 8.3

	Mg/L	Treatment
Mild	<300	Conservative
Moderate	300–700	Intravenous fluids
Severe	>700	Haemodialysis

A3.

Administration of intravenous sodium bicarbonate until a urine pH of 7.5–8.5 is reached. This increases the elimination of salicylate in the urine.

Further Reading

Toxbase.   *Bisoprolol-Fumarate.*   Available   from: https://www.toxbase.org/Poisons-Index-A-Z/S-Products/Salicylates/

SAQ 16 Tricyclic Antidepressant Toxicity

An 18-year-old female attends having taken an overdose of amitriptyline.

Q1. Give two common clinical signs associated with an amitriptyline overdose.
Q2. How is the corrected QT calculated and what is the name of this formula?
Q3. List three other causes of prolonged QT interval.

Answers

A1.

Tachycardia, mydriasis, and possibly divergent squint once obtunded. Other signs/symptoms are outlined in Table 8.4.

Table 8.4

Anticholinergic	CNS	Cardiovascular
Blurred vision	Agitation	Tachycardia
Dry mouth	Anxiety	PR prolongation
Urinary retention	Confusion	Heart block
Dilated pupils	Coma	Wide QRS, QT
Impaired sweating	Seizures	Cardiac arrest
Thermoregulation disruption	Ophthalmoplegia	Ventricular tachyarrhythmias
Various gastrointestinal effects	Rigidity	Hypotension

A2.

The most common formula used is Bazett's formula: $QT_C = QT/\sqrt{RR}$.
   NB: this is most appropriate for heart rates between 60 and 100 bpm. Other accepted formulas/answers are:

Fridericia's formula: $QT_C = QT/RR^{1/3}$
Framingham formula: $QT_C = QT + 0.154 (1—RR)$
Hodges formula: $QT_C = QT + 1.75 (heart rate—60)$

A3.

Any of the following answers are acceptable:

• Hypokalaemia
• Hypomagnesaemia
• Hypocalcaemia

- Hypothermia
- Myocardial ischaemia
- Post-cardiac arrest
- Raised intracranial pressure
- Congenital long QT syndrome
- Medication

Further Reading

Life in the Fast Lane. *Long QT Syndrome*. Available from: https://lifeinthefastlane.com/ccc/long-qt-syndrome/

Toxbase. *Amitriptyline*. Available from: https://www.toxbase.org/Poisons-Index-A-Z/A-Products/Amitriptyline----------------/

SAQ 17 **Lithium Toxicity**

A 40-year-old woman, undergoing treatment by the mental health team for manic depression, presents two hours after an overdose of slow release lithium.

Q1.   What elimination method should you consider at this stage?
Q2.   Give two physical signs you would expect to see in lithium toxicity.
Q3.   Give four other management steps in the medical treatment of this patient.

Answers

A1.

Whole bowel irrigation using polyethylene glycol is recommended for toxicity related to ingestion of sustained-release lithium. Oral activated charcoal cannot bind lithium ions.

A2.

Physical signs of lithium toxicity include tremor, ataxia, confusion, abnormal movements, increased tone, hyperreflexia and clonus, syncope, hypothermia, or hyperthermia.

A3.

Management includes:

- Intravenous fluids to maintain hydration
- Monitoring (ECG, serial neurological observations)
- Correction of electrolyte imbalance
- Measurement of serum lithium level
- Consideration of haemodialysis (in every patient with a serum lithium level greater than 4 mmol/L, irrespective of symptoms)

NB: Lithium comes as either lithium carbonate or lithium citrate. Assess all patients who have ingested more than 50 mg/kg lithium carbonate or more than 100 mg/kg lithium citrate.

Further Reading

More information about whole bowel irrigation is available from: http://emedicine.medscape.com/article/1413446-overview

Toxbase. *Lithium Citrate*. Available from: https://www.toxbase.org/Poisons-Index-A-Z/L-Products/Lithium-Citrate/

SAQ 18 **Alcohol Withdrawal**

A 45-year-old gentleman attends the emergency department after a minor fall. Your FY2 suspects this, and his previous 14 presentations this year, are related to excess alcohol consumption.

Q1. What is the name of the three-question screening tool to detect patients involved in high-risk drinking?

Q2. If you suspect the patient to be withdrawing, what scoring system would you use to identify who needs treatment?

Q3. What two pharmacological treatment would you start if you deem the patient to be withdrawing?

Answers

A1.

AUDIT-C
The questions are:

- How often do you have a drink containing alcohol?
- How many units of alcohol do you drink on a typical day when you are drinking?
- How often have you had six or more units if female, or eight or more if male, on a single occasion in the last year?

A2.

The CIWA score (Clinical Institute Withdrawal Assessment for Alcohol). The score includes assessments of nausea/vomiting, tremors, anxiety, agitation, paroxysmal sweats, orientation, tactile disturbances, auditory disturbances, visual disturbances, and headache.

A3.

Chlordiazepoxide and Pabrinex®. Thiamine supplementation (Pabrinex®) reduces the risk of Wernicke's encephalopathy. High potency injection of one pair of ampoules of Pabrinex®, mixed together, is administered by intravenous infusion in 100 ml 0.9% saline or 5% glucose over 30 minutes thrice daily for three days

Chlordiazepoxide is commenced at 10–30 mg qds orally, depending on the patient and the presentation. There is wide variation in dosing schedules, and local guidance should be followed and adhered to.

Further Reading

RCEM. *RCEM Summary of NICE Guidance CG100 (2010) & CG115 (2011)*. Available from: https://www.rcem.ac.uk/docs/External%20Guidance/10e.%20RCEM%20Summary%20of%20NICE%20CG100%20+%20CG115%20(Jan%202012).pdf

SAQ 19 **Ethylene Glycol Overdose**

A 52-year-old man is brought in by the police under section 136. He was found drinking from a bottle of antifreeze.

Q1.   What are the two main toxic substances found in antifreeze?
Q2.   How would you calculate the osmolar gap?
Q3.   How would you treat this overdose?

Answers

A1.

Ethylene glycol and methanol.

A2.

Osmolar gap = measured osmolality – calculated osmolality.
   Calculated osmolality = 2Na + glucose + urea.

A3.

Intravenous fomepizole or ethanol. Fomepizole is preferred as it has less inebriating side effects. The loading dose of fomepizole is 15 mg/kg.

Further Reading

Life in the Fast Lane. *Toxicology Conundrum*. Available from: https://lifeinthefastlane.com/toxicology-conundrum-035/

SAQ 20 **Electrocution**

A 40-year-old male is brought into the emergency department after a possible electrocution injury sustained at home while embarking on a do-it-yourself project.

Q1. List two ophthalmic conditions that frequently develop after a significant electrocution injury.

Q2. What biochemical marker would you test for to determine the severity of the electrical burden?

Q3. What other bedside test would you perform to risk stratify the patient?

Answers

A1.

Cataract and glaucoma can develop following an electrical injury. Other injuries are corneal burns, retinal detachment, and intraocular haemorrhage.

A2.

Creatine kinase is a useful marker of severity, being released by the damaged skeletal muscle tissue.

A3.

Urine dipstick: a positive urine dip for blood but with little or no red blood cells on microscopy would indicate the presence of myoglobinuria.

Further Reading

RCEM Learning. *Electrical Injuries*. Available from: https://www.rcemlearning.co.uk/references/electrical-injuries/

Chapter 9 **Gastroenterology**

SAQ 1 **Hepatitis A**

The triage note for your next patient says '19 Male, thinks he has turned into Homer Simpson, generally unwell'. Amused by your triage nurse's choice of wording, you take a history from the visibly jaundiced gentleman. He has been feeling unwell for over a week with fatigue, general aches, nausea, and abdominal discomfort. The past few days he has become icteric, his urine has darkened, and stools have become pale. He returned from travelling around Southeast Asia 5 weeks previously. Hepatitis A is top of your differential diagnoses.

Q1. Apart from foreign travel, list two other risk factors to ask the patient about in order to assess his risk for hepatitis.
Q2. Which serological result would indicate an acute infection?
Q3. Give one scenario which would mandate the immediate reporting of this patient's suspected hepatitis A to the Health Protection Agency.

Answers

A1.

Any of the following are indicative of hepatitis risk (list two):

- Clotting disorders (risk of contaminated blood products)
- Sexual practice involving oral–anal or digital–rectal contact, group sex, sex in public places, multiple sexual partners, men having sex with men
- Injecting drug use (including close contacts)
- Occupational risk: laboratory workers, residential institution workers, sewage workers, those working with primates

A2.

Positive HAV-specific IgM antibodies would suggest an acute infection and are detectable 1–2 weeks after the onset of symptoms for approximately three months.

Positive HAV-IgG antibodies, although present in acute infection (around 5–10 days after infection), do not allow differentiation of acute from past infection.

A3.

If either, the patient is a food handler or the patient's case is part of a suspected outbreak, immediate reporting is mandated.

Hepatitis A is a self-limiting illness, presenting with non-specific prodromal systemic symptoms, such as anorexia, malaise, fever, nausea, followed by abdominal symptoms, such as abdominal discomfort or pain, jaundice, pruritus, and dark urine (due to bilirubinuria).

Further Reading

NICE. *Hepatitis A—NICE CKS*. 2014. Available from: http://cks.nice.org.uk/hepatitis-a

SAQ 2 **Spontaneous Bacterial Peritonitis**

A 43-year-old man suffering with alcohol dependence presents to the emergency department with confusion, lethargy, and altered affect. You notice his abdomen is very swollen—his family say this is getting worse. You discuss with your medical colleagues as you think this man is at risk of having spontaneous bacterial peritonitis (SBP).

Q1. What is the most common pathogen causing SBP?
Q2. How is the diagnosis of SBP made?
Q3. Which are the two most common presenting symptoms?

Answers

A1.

Escherichia coli is the most common causative agent of SBP; other organisms include other coliforms (such as *Klebsiella pneumoniae*) and *Streptococcus pneumoniae*. This makes third-generation cephalosporins, such as cefotaxime, ceftriaxone, and ceftazidime, the antibiotics of choice for initial treatment.

A2.

The diagnosis is made by finding an absolute neutrophil count (ANC) of more than 250 cells/mm^3 on ascitic tap, associated with a subsequent positive bacterial culture, in the absence of any obvious evidence of intra-abdominal and potentially surgically treatable source of infection (such as visceral inflammation or perforation).

A3.

Fever (often with chills) and diffuse abdominal pain are the most common presenting symptoms. Other symptoms include vomiting and increased confusion.

NB: The importance of early diagnosis makes this a relevant topic for the emergency physician as prompt ascitic tap can be invaluable. Those with hepatic encephalopathy, decompensated liver cirrhosis, higher than usual ascites volume and/or frequency of accumulation, history of gastrointestinal bleeding, and those who have had recent endoscopy are at an especially elevated risk for SBP. Although clinical findings can be useful, they are not reliable; therefore, even those seemingly at low risk of SBP should have an ascitic tap as part of the workup to rule it out. Ascitic cultures are negative in up to 60% of SBP, hence the diagnostic criterion is a raised neutrophil count in tap.

Further Reading

BMJ Best Practice. *Spontaneous Bacterial Peritonitis*. Available from: http://bestpractice.bmj.com/best-practice/monograph/793.html
EASL. *Management of Ascites, Spontaneous Bacterial Peritonitis, and Hepatorenal Syndrome in Cirrhosis*. 2010. Available from: https://easl.eu/wp-content/uploads/2018/10/Hepatorenal-Cirrhosis-English-report.pdf

SAQ 3 **Acute Pancreatitis**

A 57-year-old male presents with acute upper abdominal pain, anorexia, nausea, and vomiting. He has a history of alcohol abuse.

Q1. What is the likely presenting differential diagnosis? List two.
Q2. List the chemical markers used to determine severity of acute pancreatitis (at least four).
Q3. What investigations confirm a diagnosis of acute pancreatitis? List two.

Answers

A1.

The most likely initial diagnoses to consider include acute pancreatitis or alcoholic gastritis.

A2.

The Glasgow modified acute pancreatitis severity score (Imrie's criteria) lists the following markers of severity of acute pancreatitis:

- PaO$_2$ <8.0 kPa
- Age >55 years
- WBC count >15 × 10 ^9/L
- Serum calcium <2 mmol/L
- Urea >16 mmol/L
- LDH >600 IU/L; AST >2000 IU/L
- Albumin <32 g/L
- Glucose >10 mmol/L

Severe pancreatitis is defined by the presence of more than three criteria within 48 hours of presentation.

A3.

The diagnosis of acute pancreatitis is confirmed by:

- Serum lipase or amylase elevation more than three times upper limit of normal.
- Characteristic imaging features on contrast-enhanced abdominal computed tomography (CT), MRI, or ultrasound, which include focal or diffuse enlargement of the pancreas, homogeneous or heterogenous enhancement of the parenchyma, ill-defined pancreatic margins, and retroperitoneal fat stranding.
- Contrast-enhanced CT can also detect pancreatic necrosis and peripancreatic fluid collections.

Further Reading

Blamey SL, Imrie CW, O' Neill SJ, Gilmour WH, Carter DC. Prognostic factors in acute pancreatitis. *Gut.* 1984;25:1340–6.

BSG. Available at: http://www.bsg.org.uk/images/stories/docs/clinical/guidelines/pancreatic/pancreatic.pdf

NICE. *Pancreatitis—Acute*. Available at: https://cks.nice.org.uk/pancreatitis-acute#!scenario

SAQ 4 **Upper Gastrointestinal Bleeding**

A 45-year-old man presents following two episodes of vomiting blood, which appear to have settled. Your FY2 trainee would like to discharge him but is unsure on how to risk stratify the patient.

Q1. What two risk assessment scores are you aware of and which one is more useful in the emergency department?

Q2. After 15 minutes in the resuscitation room, the nurse in charge walks in and tells you she knows the patient well, he attends almost daily due to chronic alcohol abuse and is well known to the gastroenterology team for his oesophageal varices. What treatment could you start to reduce his bleeding (route and dosage)?

Q3. If medication alone is unable alone to control presumed variceal bleeding, what medical device would you consider?

Answers

A1.

The Blatchford score and the Rockall score.

Both are risk assessment scores for upper gastrointestinal (GI) bleeding. The Blatchford score can be calculated in the ED and a patient with a score of 0 could be suitable for outpatient endoscopy follow-up. The Rockall score depends on findings of endoscopy and hence is not that useful at first presentation to the ED. The features of the Blatchford score and the Rockall score are outlined in Table 9.1.

Table 9.1

Blatchford score	Rockall score
Haemoglobin level (G/L)	Age (years)
Urea (mmol/L)	Shock
Systolic blood pressure (mm Hg)	Comorbidities
Heart rate (>==100 bpm)	Endoscopy results (diagnosis)
Melaena	Stigmata of bleed (on endoscopy)
Syncope	
Hepatic disease	
Cardiac failure	

A2.

Administration of 2 g intravenous terlipressin is the first-line management. This acts as a vasocon-strictor, alternative treatments are somatostatin, or octreotide (unlicensed).

Antibiotics are recommended for all patients with suspected or confirmed variceal bleeding. Consider blood product replacement as per local massive transfusion protocol.

A3.

Use of a Sengstaken–Blakemore tube. This has three lumens, one for inflation of a gastric balloon, one for inflation of an oesophageal balloon, and one for aspiration of gastric contents. In most patients, initially only the gastric balloon is inflated, followed by inflation of the oesophageal balloon in the case of continued variceal bleeding,

Further Reading

Blatchford O, Murray WR, Blatchford M. A risk score to predict need for treatment for upper gastrointestinal haemorrhage. *Lancet.* 2000;356(9238):1318–21.
Tripathi D, Stanley AJ, Hayes PC, Patch D, Millson C, Mehrzad H, et al. UK guidelines on the management of variceal haemorrhage in cirrhotic patients. *Gut.* 2015;64:1680–704.

SAQ 5 **Ulcerative Colitis**

A 32-year-old male with a 4-year history of ulcerative colitis attends the ED with a history of bloody diarrhoea.

Q1. List four criteria for assessing severity of the presentation.
Q2. List treatment priorities for a severe attack.
Q3. What acute abdominal complications should be considered? List three

Answers

A1.

Any of the following are indicative of severity:

- Number of bowel movements per day
- Presence of blood in the stools
- Temperature more than 37.8°C
- Pulse rate more than 90 bpm
- Anaemia
- ESR more than 30 mm/hour

These are known as the Truelove and Witts' severity index, which allows recognition of three categories: mild, moderate, or severe.

A2.

The following are acceptable answers:

- Multidisciplinary team management, including gastroenterologist and colorectal surgeon, and a paediatrician if the patient is a child and an obstetrician for a pregnant patient
- Intravenous corticosteroids
- Consideration of intravenous ciclosporin or surgery

A3.

Abdominal complications of ulcerative colitis include:

- Colonic dilatation (toxic megacolon), which is recognized by plain radiography of the abdomen, when the transverse colon is dilated to at least 6 cm
- Fulminant colitis
- Bowel perforation
- Stricture of the bowel

Further Reading

NICE. *Ulcerative Colitis: Management CG166*. Available from: https://www.nice.org.uk/guidance/cg166/chapter/1-Recommendations#maintaining-remission-in-people-with-ulcerative-colitis

SAQ 6 **Anaemia**

A young non-pregnant lady comes in complaining of feeling tired all the time. She says she cannot wait for a GP appointment. Her full blood count shows microcytic anaemia.

Q1. Below what value would her result be considered anaemia?

Q2. What test will you recommend her GP to do to detect iron deficiency anaemia?

Q3. What features would prompt you to consider admitting her and/or transfusing acutely?

Answers

A1.

Haemoglobin below 12 g/dl defines anaemia in non-pregnant women over 15 years of age. The World Health Organization (WHO) criteria further define anaemia as haemoglobin level below 13 g/dl in men over 15 years of age, and below 12 g/dl in children aged 12 to 14 years.

A2.

Serum ferritin level.

This correlates best with total body iron stores in the body. However, it can be raised as an in-flammatory marker and so caution needs to be taken when finding this as 'normal', as high levels can coexist with iron deficiency anaemia in the presence of infection or inflammation. Some conditions which often cause a raised ferritin are rheumatoid disease, liver disease, malignancy, hyperthyroidism, kidney disease, and heavy alcohol use. Other inflammatory markers will probably also be somewhat raised.

A3.

Angina, marked ankle oedema, or dyspnoea at rest.

All are suggestive of impact on cardiac function and may prompt immediate management as these may be evidence of acute and ongoing blood loss alongside the known anaemia.

Further Reading

NICE. *Anaemia—Iron Deficiency—NICE CKS*. 2013. Available from: https://cks.nice.org.uk/anaemia-iron-deficiency#!topicsummary

SAQ 7 **Haemorrhoids**

A 34-year-old lady presents, complaining of lots of pain from her 'piles'. You find a cubicle and a colleague to chaperone while you examine her.

Q1. What findings might prompt you to admit this lady acutely under the surgeons?
Q2. What are the options for topical treatment?
Q3. What would be your advice on topical treatment if she is pregnant or breastfeeding?

Answers

A1.

Complications of haemorrhoids requiring surgical referral include:

- External haemorrhoids which are thrombosed acutely, exquisitely painful, and have presented within 72 hours of onset (they may benefit from reduction and excision)
- Prolapsed internal haemorrhoids which are swollen, thrombosed, and incarcerated (this may be an indication for haemorrhoidectomy)
- Evidence of perianal sepsis (this, although rare, can be life-threatening)

A2.

Mild astringents or lubricants can be effective at relieving local irritation.

Local anaesthetic creams can cause skin sensitization; however, they may alleviate the burning, pain, and itching (lidocaine is the least irritant choice of the anaesthetic agents).

Agents with corticosteroids may also help with pain and inflammation; however, they can cause skin atrophy, contact dermatitis, or skin sensitization. Local infections must be ruled out before use.

A3.

There is no topical product which is licensed for use in either pregnancy or breastfeeding women; however, if one must be used, advise one without local anaesthetic or corticosteroids.

Further Reading

NICE. *Haemorrhoids—NICE CKS*. 2016. Available from: https://cks.nice.org.uk/haemorrhoids#!scenario

Chapter 10 **Haematology**

SAQ 1 **Henoch–Schönlein Purpura**

A 10-year-old boy attends the emergency department complaining of colicky abdominal pain and a rash on the legs, which his mother tested for blanching. The rash started the previous day and the abdominal pain the same morning. The parents mentioned that he had been seen by his general practitioner in the preceding week for a bad 'chest cold' and was treated with paracetamol. The non-blanching rash is limited to the legs and buttock area.

Q1. What is your working diagnosis?
Q2. What other clinical features can occur? List three.
Q3. How is this condition managed?

Answers

A1.

Henoch–Schönlein purpura is suggested by the combination of abdominal pain and skin rash.

A2.

Other clinical features include polyarthralgia or haematuria. The disease begins with the sudden onset of a palpable purpuric rash that typically involves the extensor surfaces of the feet, legs, and arms, and a strip across the buttocks. The purpura may start as small areas of urticaria that become indurated and palpable. Crops of new lesions may appear over days to several weeks. Many patients also have fever and polyarthralgia with associated periarticular tenderness and swelling of the ankles, knees, hips, wrists, and elbows. Gastrointestinal manifestations are common and include colicky abdominal pain, abdominal tenderness, and melena. Intussusception occasionally develop, leading to small bowel obstruction. The stool may test positive for occult blood. Symptoms usually remit after about 4 weeks but often recur at least once after a disease-free interval of several weeks. In most patients, the disorder subsides without serious sequelae.

A3.

The management is mainly supportive, with occasionally the need for oral corticosteroids, as the condition is mostly self-limited.

The clinical diagnosis is confirmed by biopsy of skin lesions, with identification of leukocytoclastic vasculitis with IgA in the vessel walls. Haematuria, proteinuria, and red blood cell casts indicate kidney involvement. Renal biopsy should be obtained if renal function is deteriorating and may help define the prognosis. Diffuse glomerular involvement or crescentic changes in most glomeruli predict progressive renal failure.

Corticosteroids help in symptomatic control of joint pains and abdominal pain, but not with coexisting renal impairment. Immunosuppressive therapy may be required for those with severe renal impairment.

Further Reading

Vasculitis UK. *IgA Vasculitis (Henoch-Schönlein Purpura)*. Available from: http://www.vasculitis.org.uk/about-vasculitis/henoch-schonlein-purpura

SAQ 2 Immune Thrombocytopenia

A 15-year-old female, who is generally fit and well, presents with a petechial rash and epistaxis following a recent viral upper respiratory infection. She is not on any medication and is haemodynamically stable. On examination, she is apyrexial and there is no lymphadenopathy or hepatosplenomegaly.

Q1. What is the most likely diagnosis?
Q2. What findings might be expected on blood tests (list two)?
Q3. What treatment options are available for this condition (list three)?

Answers

A1.

The most likely diagnosis is idiopathic thrombocytopenic purpura (immune thrombocytopenia).

A2.

Blood tests typically show the following:

- Platelet count <100 000/cu mm
- Normal white cell and red cell count (anaemia may occur in the presence of significant bleeding)
- Isolated thrombocytopenia is characteristic of idiopathic thrombocytopenic purpura

A3.

The options depend on disease severity and include:

- Watchful expectancy; with no bleeding or mild bleeding (skin manifestations alone) can be managed with observation alone, irrespective of actual platelet count
- Steroid therapy
- Immunosuppression: rituximab, azathioprine, cyclophosphamide
- Intravenous immunoglobulin; anti-D immunoglobulin
- Splenectomy

Further Reading

Neunert C, Lim W, Crowther M, Cohen A, Solberg L Jr, Crowther MA, et al. The American Society of Hematology 2011 evidence-based practice guideline for immune thrombocytopenia. *Blood*. 2011;117(16):4190–207.

SAQ 3 **Sickle Cell Crisis**

A 22-year-old female, known to have sickle cell disease, attends the emergency department with severe generalized body ache, similar to previous presentations to the emergency department. She is apyrexial and her vital signs are stable, including an SpO_2 of 98%.

Q1. List two important treatment priorities in the emergency department.
Q2. What complications should be looked for in an acute crisis? List four.
Q3. What is the role of oxygen therapy?

Answers

A1.

Two important priorities are:

1. Analgesia, titrated to pain severity. Severe pain usually mandates opiate therapy, morphine 0.1 mg/kg intravenous, repeated every 20 minutes until pain is relieved. Many patients have a personal treatment plan and named haematologist. Treatment should be guided by these if available. Patient-controlled analgesia may be necessary if repeated opiate boluses are required within a two-hour period.
2. Rehydration, which may be oral or intravenous.

A2.

An acute crisis can be complicated by any of the following:

- Infection
- Acute chest syndrome (acute respiratory symptoms and new infiltrate on chest X-ray)
- Aplastic crisis
- Splenic sequestration
- Priapism
- Stroke
- Osteomyelitis

A3.

Oxygen should not be routinely administered. An SpO_2 of 92% or less indicates the need for oxygen therapy, guided by continuous pulse oximetry and serial arterial blood gases.

Further Reading

NICE. *Sickle Cell Disease: Managing Acute Painful Episodes in Hospital CG143*. 2012. Available from: https://www.nice.org.uk/guidance/cg143

US Department of Health Expert Panel Report. 2014. Available from: https://www.nhlbi.nih.gov/sites/default/files/media/docs/sickle-cell-disease-report%20020816_0.pdf

SAQ 4 **Haemolytic Transfusion Reaction**

A 65-year-old man is receiving a blood transfusion for upper gastrointestinal bleeding while in the emergency department awaiting endoscopy. He complains of back and chest pain, dizziness, and shortness of breath. His vital signs are: heart rate 110 bpm, blood pressure 80/60 mm Hg, respiratory rate 24/minute, temperature 37.5°C.

Q1. What is the most likely diagnosis?
Q2. List four important actions in the emergency department.
Q3. What measures could help prevent recurrence of this episode (list two)?

Answers

A1.

Acute intravascular haemolytic transfusion reaction is the most likely diagnosis and needs to be considered as a priority. The symptoms are often non-specific, due to rapid red cell destruction (of either, or both, the patient's and the transfused red cells), developing during or within 24 hours of blood transfusion. Other clinical features may include agitation, a burning sensation at the infusion site and along the vein receiving the infusion, headache, nausea, vomiting, fever and chills, skin changes, tachycardia, tachypnoea, hypotension, and red urine (haemoglobinuria).

A2.

In the emergency department, the following interventions should be initiated:

- Stop the transfusion.
- Intravenous crystalloid infusion, with or without diuretic (e.g. furosemide), to initiate diuresis of at least 100 ml/hour.
- Check documentation, including patient identity and all transfused units.
- Take blood for testing.
- Urine testing for haemoglobin.
- Return all transfused packs to the transfusion laboratory.
- Incident reporting to allow for thorough investigation of the root causes underlying the incident. The Serious Hazards of Transfusion (SHOT) UK confidential haemo-vigilance reporting scheme, which commenced in 1996, has allowed for improvements in transfusion safety.

A3.

Haemolytic transfusion reactions can be prevented by:

- Double checking of all transfusion documentation (mislabelling of patient samples and of blood products is the major factor in causation)
- Bar-coded samples and blood packs

Further Reading

British Society for Haematology. *Investigation and Management of Acute Transfusion Reactions*. 2012. Available from: http://www.b-s-h.org.uk/guidelines/guidelines/investigation-and-management-of-acute-transfusion-reactions/

SAQ 5 **Over-anticoagulation**

A 79-year-old male is brought to the resuscitation room with an altered level of consciousness. A CT scan of the head shows an acute subdural haematoma. He is noted to be on warfarin for atrial fibrillation, and his international normalized ratio (INR) is 7.

Q1. What measures should you consider to manage the INR? List two.
Q2. List four pharmacological prohaemostatic agents that can be used for managing significant bleeding related to therapy with antithrombotic agents.
Q3. Name three novel oral anticoagulant drugs, along with their mode of action.

Answers

A1.

In the presence of life-threatening haemorrhage and a grossly prolonged INR, management comprises:

- Vitamin K 1 mg slow intravenous
- Four-factor prothrombin complex concentrate containing factors II, VII, IX, and X at dose of 50 IU factor IX or factor VII per kg body weight
- If no concentrate is available,1 litre fresh frozen plasma should be infused in an adult

A2.

Prohaemostatic agents that may be useful in an emergency include:

- Tranexamic acid
- Desmopressin
- Fresh frozen plasma
- Cryoprecipitate
- Platelet transfusion
- Prothrombin complex concentrate

A3.

Novel oral anticoagulant drugs in current use include:

- Apixaban: direct inhibitor of Factor Xa
- Rivaroxaban: direct inhibitor of Factor Xa
- Dabigatran: direct inhibitor of thrombin

Further Reading

British Society for Haematology. Management of bleeding in patients on antithrombotic agents. *British Journal of Haematology*. 2013;160:35–46.

SAQ 6 Management of Jehovah's Witness Potentially Requiring Blood Transfusion

A 36-year-old female has been brought to the resuscitation room, with multiple trauma and a splenic injury, for which surgical intervention is likely to be required owing to haemodynamic instability. You are informed that she is a Jehovah's witness and will not accept a blood transfusion under any circumstances. She has an Advance Decision document.

Q1.   What options do you have for haemodynamic support?
Q2.   What intraoperative options are available?
Q3.   What specific actions might be required for this patient? List three.

Answers

A1.

It is important to respect the views of an adult patient in the presence of adequate capacity, even if death is a possible outcome of refusal of treatment. An Advance Directive is legally binding. Jehovah's Witnesses' interpretation of the Bible lead to their refusal of whole blood transfusions. The options include:

- The use of crystalloid solutions such as normal saline and Hartmann's solution to replace volume losses, aiming for normovolaemic haemodilution
- Autologous blood transfusion

A2.

Most Jehovah's Witnesses will accept extracorporeal equipment and procedures using their own blood, such as intraoperative cell salvage for blood conservation. In the appropriate situations, cardiopulmonary bypass using a non-blood fluid prime for the heart–lung machine is acceptable.

A3.

Options available for individual patients include:

- Contacting the Hospital Liaison Committee for Jehovah's Witnesses to help coordinate patient care
- Use of antifibrinolytic drugs, such as intravenous tranexamic acid
- Discussion with individual patients the acceptability of plasma derivatives (prothrombin complex concentrate) and cryoprecipitate
- Good haemostatic technique, including use of topical haemostatic agents (including fibrin glue and thrombin gel), involving the principles of 'bloodless surgery'
- Initiating postoperative iron replacement. Erythropoeitin has also been recommended in this situation.

Further Reading

British Committee for Standards in Haematology Guidelines (BCSH). *Caring for Patients Who Refuse Blood: A Guide to Good Practice for Management of Jehovah's Witnesses and Other Patients Who Decline Transfusion*. London, UK: Royal College of Surgeons of England, November 2016. Available from: https://www.rcseng.ac.uk/-/media/files/rcs/library-and-publications/non-journal-publications/caring-for-patients-who-refuse-blood--a-guide-to-good-practice.pdf

Chapter 11 **Infectious Diseases**

SAQ 1 **Acute Epiglottitis**

A 48-year-old male is brought in with difficulty in breathing and stridor. Ambulance personnel have given him intramuscular adrenaline and nebulized salbutamol with no effect. He is struggling to breathe, and keeps saying 'I'm dying'. He is febrile (39°C), tachycardic (120 beats per minute), and hypotensive (90/60 mm Hg). He has no known allergies.

Q1.   Give three possible differential diagnoses.
Q2.   What is your management plan (list three)?
Q3.   Describe the landmarks and technique for a surgical airway.

Answers

A1.

Any three of the following should be considered:

- Acute epiglottitis
- Quinsy
- Ludwig's angina
- Retropharyngeal abscess
- Anaphylaxis
- Foreign body

A2.

The management of suspected acute epiglottitis includes:

- Move to the resuscitation room
- Keep the patient calm and sat upright. Do not attempt visualization of the epiglottis with a tongue depressor
- Intravenous broad-spectrum antibiotics—ceftriaxone 2 g
- Hydrocortisone 100 mg intravenous

A senior anaesthetist and an ear, nose, throat (ENT) surgeon should be contacted for airway management. If possible, the patient should be intubated in the operating theatre with gas induction.

A3.

- Feel for gap between cricoid and thyroid membrane (cricothyroid membrane)
- Make horizontal incision to skin, down to and through cricothyroid membrane

- Once through the membrane, turn the scalpel 90 degrees (sharp end to feet)
- Pass bougie through hole alongside scalpel
- Railroad tracheal tube over bougie

Further Reading

Difficult Airway Society. *DAS Guidelines For Management Of Unanticipated Difficult Intubation In Adults 2015.* 2015. Available from: https://www.das.uk.com/guidelines/das_intubation_guidelines

SAQ 2 **Meningitis**

Jo, a 22-year-old medical student, is brought in by his flatmate. He has been complaining of a fever and headache. He is febrile 38°C. The triage nurse gives him some paracetamol and sends him to the walk-in centre next door. About 15 minutes later, you are called to the urgent care centre as he had a seizure in the waiting area. On your arrival, he is on the floor with a Glasgow Coma Score of E 2 V 3 M 4.

Q1. What is the most likely diagnosis, and list the common causative organisms in this population?

Q2. Outline your immediate management, including treatment specific to this diagnosis.

Q3. Jimmy and Matt are Jo's flatmates—they are worried that they may catch what Jo had. What prophylaxis can you offer?

Answers

A1.

In meningitis, common causative bacteria are:

- *Neisseria meningitidis*
- *Haemophilus influenzae B*
- *Streptococcus pneumoniae*
- Listeria
- *Cryptococcus*
- Herpes

A2.

Transfer to the resuscitation room and initiate the following:

- Secure airway
- Resuscitate with fluids
- Ceftriaxone 2 g IV
- Consider aciclovir
- Computed tomography (CT) brain
- Polymerase chain reaction testing for bacterial antigen
- Consider lumbar puncture depending on presence or absence of signs of raised intracranial pressure.

A3.

Rifampicin or ciprofloxacin are recommended for meningococcal chemoprophylaxis. Ciprofloxacin is recommended in all age groups and in pregnancy, and is advantageous as it is given as a single dose.

NB: Rifampicin covers haemophilus influenzae type B and Neisseria meningitidis. Consider giving prophylaxis to all household or childcare contacts, as well as clinicians exposed to upper airway secretions.

Further Reading

Meningitis Research Foundation. *Resources for Health Professionals and Their Patients.* Available from: http://www. meningitis.org/health-professionals/hospital-protocols-adults

SAQ 3 **HIV Post-exposure Prophylaxis**

A 32-year-old male ward nurse attends the emergency department following a needle stick injury sustained to his left index finger while he was obtaining a venous blood sample. The patient he was bleeding is HIV positive.

Q1. What factors increase the risk of HIV transmission in this situation?
Q2. What initial management is recommended?
Q3. What specific treatment is indicated in this situation?

Answers

A1.

The potential risk of HIV transmission is increased by:

- Visible blood contamination of the needle
- Needle placement in the patient's vein
- Use of a large hollow-bore needle

It is worth noting that a range of bodily fluids other than blood may be associated with the risk of transmission of HIV infection, including blood-stained saliva, cerebrospinal, amniotic, rectal, peritoneal, synovial, pericardial, or pleural fluids, as well as breast milk and genital secretions.

A2.

Initial management in this situation includes:

- Washing of the wound under running water
- Encourage active bleeding
- Venous blood is taken for baseline hepatitis B, C, and HIV status with consent

A3.

Post-exposure prophylaxis, usually triple-therapy antiretroviral therapy, should be considered. Advice from the microbiology department and the occupational health service is recommended. An HIV-positive donor with an undetectable plasma viral load may not always warrant recipient prophylaxis in this situation.

Further Reading

BHIVA. *UK National Guideline for the Use of HIV Post-Exposure Prophylaxis Following Sexual Exposure (PEPSE).* 2015. Available from: http://www.bhiva.org/PEPSE-guidelines.aspx

SAQ 4 **Neutropenic Sepsis**

You are reviewing your department's guidance for adult neutropenic sepsis:

Q1. What is the definition of neutropenic sepsis?
Q2. What puts a patient at risk of neutropenia?
Q3. List the components of the sepsis 6 care bundle?

Answers

A1.

The National Institute for Health and Care Excellence (NICE)-recognized definition for neutropenic sepsis is:
38°C temperature OR any signs/symptoms of sepsis* AND a neutrophil count of 0.5×10^9/L or less

*Sepsis is defined as a life-threatening organ dysfunction caused by a dysregulated host response to an infection. Historically, the SIRS (**S**ystemic **I**nflammatory **R**esponse **S**yndrome) criteria were used to identify patients at high risk of sepsis (>2 of the following 4 criteria):

Temperature >38°C or <36°C
Heart rate >90/minute
Respiratory rate >20/minute
White blood cell count $>12 \times 10^9$/L or $<4.0 \times 10^9$/L

The SIRS criteria are now thought to be neither sensitive nor specific. A newer scoring system has been devised: SOFA (**S**equential **O**rgan **F**ailure **A**ssessment). This scoring system is believed to be more specific but requires more biochemical markers and takes into account the requirement of vasopressors to predict mortality. In the emergency department, the abbreviate qSOFA (**q**uick **S**equential **O**rgan **F**ailure **A**ssessment) can be used to predict which patient are more likely to have a poor outcome: Glasgow coma score of less than 15, respiratory rate more than 22 /minute, or hypotension (systolic blood pressure <100 mm Hg). The presence of more than two out of the three predicts poor outcome.

A2.

Any from the following list can put someone at risk of being neutropenic:
HIV, TB, overwhelming bacterial sepsis, viral infection (e.g. varicella, measles, EBV, CMV), cytotoxic chemotherapy, bone marrow transplant, disease-modifying antirheumatic drugs, carbimazole, clozapine/olanzapine, B_{12}/folate deficiency, aplastic anaemia, myelodysplasia, leukaemia, paroxysmal nocturnal haemoglobinuria, hypersplenism, congenital neutropenia, white-cell aplasia, reticular dysgenesis, dyskeratosis congenita, Chédiak–Higashi syndrome.

A3.

The following steps constitute the sepsis 6:

- Give intravenous antibiotics
- Give intravenous fluids
- Give high-flow oxygen
- Take blood cultures
- Take (monitor) urine output
- Take lactate

NB: you give three and you take three.

Further Reading

NICE. *Neutropenic Sepsis: Prevention and Management in People with Cancer 2012, CG151.* Available from: https://www.nice.org.uk/guidance/cg151

qSOFA. *Quick Sepsis Related Organ Failure Assessment.* Available from: http://www.qsofa.org

Singer M, Deutschman CS, Seymour CW, Shankar-Hari M, Annane D, Bauer M, et al. The Third International Consensus Definitions for Sepsis and Septic Shock (Sepsis-3). *JAMA.* 2016;315(8):801–10.

SAQ 5 Ebola Virus Infection

Your department has been made vigilant once again for cases of possible Ebola virus as a new epidemic is re-emerging in West Africa. You have been made responsible for ensuring appropriate safeguards are in place in your department for receiving a suspected case.

Q1. What are the two initial screening questions required to isolate possible cases of Ebola?
Q2. The Advisory Committee on Dangerous Pathogens (ACDP) advises a list of seven minimum personal protective equipment (PPE) required for entering the isolation room, what are these?
Q3. What is the mode of transmission of Ebola virus?

Answers

A1.

Has the patient been in an affected area, or cared for an Ebola case within the last 21 days?
   AND
   Does the patient have a history consistent with fever in the past 24 hours?
   Such patients ought to be isolated to a single room with facilities for hand-washing, toileting, using the phone, and placing secure kit in the bin.

A2.

There should be nine packs of PPE available, in a variety of sizes. There should also be enough PPE equipment available to manage a patient for a duration of 12 hours.
   The PPE packs should contain:

- double gloves with extra-long cuffs
- fluid repellent single use coveralls consistent with the current ACDP guidance
- ankle-length endoscopy apron
- surgical cap
- full face shield (visor)
- close fitting fluid repellent mask
- wellingtons

Further to the PPE there should be two ready-made treatment packs, containing: fluids, paracetamol, vomit bowls, absorbent granules, bin-bags with ties, phlebotomy/cannulation/peripheral line equipment.

A3.

Ebola virus is transmitted by direct contact, through broken skin or mucous membranes (e.g. eyes, nose, or mouth), with blood or body fluids (including saliva, sweat, urine, faeces, vomit, breast milk, or semen) of an infected person. Family members and healthcare workers are especially at risk of acquisition of infection.

Further Reading

RCEM. *EBOLA Guidance for Emergency Departments.* 2014. Available from: https://www.rcem.ac.uk/docs/College%20Guidelines/5a.%20Ebola%20guidance%20for%20emergency%20department.pdf

SAQ 6 **Lyme Disease**

A 35-year-old woman attends the department concerned that she has been feeling generally unwell since being bitten by 'some sort of bug' during a holiday in Exmoor one week ago. You examine her and find a 12 cm round, pink, macular rash with clearing in the centre, in the crease of her left knee.

Q1. What name is given to this rash and which disease is it likely to be associated with in this case?

Q2. Given that this lady is symptomatic of your suspected diagnosis, what would be your first-line treatment?

Q3. You mention the case to your colleague, who read up about this recently and reminds you to check whether she is pregnant or breastfeeding, in which case second-line treatment is needed. Your colleague also suggests you advise your patient to look out for a Jarisch–Herxheimer reaction after starting antibiotics, which happens in 15% of people. What is a Jarisch–Herxheimer reaction?

Answers

A1.

Erythema migrans, which appears around the site of the Ixodes tick bite, transmits the Borrelia burgdorferi bacteria. In the presence of this rash, treatment is indicated, and laboratory confirmation of infection is not required.

A2.

Oral doxycycline 100 mg bd for 14–21 days is usually advised. Amoxicillin and cefuroxime are alternative treatments.

A3.

A Jarisch–Herxheimer reaction arises due to release of toxins following bacterial death.
  It may involve:

- worsening of fever
- chills
- muscle pains
- headache
- tachycardia
- hyperventilation
- vasodilation with flushing
- mild hypotension

Usually this happens within the first 24 hours of treatment and lasts up to 2 days. If it is mild and has no evidence of allergic reaction such as urticarial, then it can be waited out and antibiotics continued. It can occur in other diseases being treated by antibiotics such as syphilis, leptospirosis, and Q fever.

Further Reading

NICE. *Lyme Disease*. NG95, 2018. Available from: https://cks.nice.org.uk/lyme-disease#!topicsummary

SAQ 7 **Dog Bite**

A 34-year-old lady attends the emergency department after sustaining a stray dog bite to her right forearm.

Q1. Give three characteristics of tetanus-prone wounds.
Q2. What treatment would you initiate in the emergency department related to tetanus status in a tetanus-prone wound if the patient has not had the full immunization programme?
Q3. If the bite had occurred in a country with a high risk of rabies, what treatment would you need to ensure has occurred on the day of the bite?

Answers

A1.

Any three of the following indicate a tetanus-prone wound:

- Heavy contamination (soil, manure)
- Wounds with foreign body
- The presence of devitalized tissue
- Wounds that require intervention or wounds older than 6 hours
- Animal bite

A2.

Give a booster dose of tetanus vaccine plus a dose of human antitetanus immunoglobulin (HATI) at a different anatomical site.

A3.

Passive immunization needs to be initiated by rabies immunoglobulin (either human or equine rabies immunoglobulin) just prior to or shortly after the first dose of rabies vaccine. A total of five doses of vaccines need to be administered: days 0, 3, 7, 14, and 28. This treatment should be conducted with guidance from the Rabies and Immunoglobulin Service, Public Health England, Colindale (020 8327 6204).

Rabies has not been diagnosed in terrestrial animals in the United Kingdom since 1922.

Further Reading

WHO. *Rabies vaccines and immunoglobulins, 2018*. Available from http://www.who.int/ith/vaccines/rabies/en/

SAQ 8 **Human Bite**

A 28-year-old police officer attends the emergency department after being bitten on his left hand, sustained while intervening in a fight. He is up to date with his immunisations but has been asked by his superior to 'get checked out'.

Q1. In order to wash the wound, you consider doing a wrist block. What anatomical landmarks can you use to perform a median nerve block?
Q2. What is the current recommendation regarding antibiotic treatment for a human bite?
Q3. He asks you about post-exposure prophylaxis (PEP). What are his risks of contracting HIV and should he start?

Answers

A1.

Palmaris longus and flexor carpi ulnaris. The nerve lies deep and radial to palmaris longus and medial to the flexor carpi ulnaris.

A2.

Current evidence suggests starting antibiotics (co-amoxiclav or metronidazole + doxycycline) for any wound less than 72 hours even if no signs of infections are noted.

A3.

The risk of HIV transmission from a known HIV-positive patient during a bite has been estimated to be less than 1/10 000, and unless there are special circumstances, it is not recommended to commence PEP.

Further Reading

NICE. *Bites—Human and Animal.* Available from: https://cks.nice.org.uk/bites-human-and-animal#!scenarioclar ification:2

UK Guideline for the use of HIV Post-Exposure Prophylaxis Following Sexual Exposure (PEPSE). 2015. Available from: https://www.bashh.org/documents/PEPSE%202015%20guideline%20final_NICE.pdf

SAQ 9 **Paronychia**

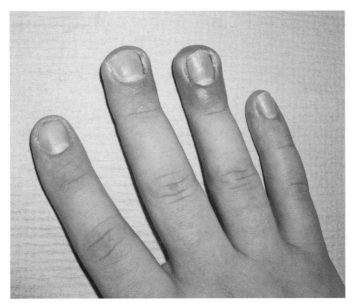

Fig. 11.1 Reproduced from Burge, S., Matin, R. and Wallis, D. (2016). *Oxford Handbook of Medical Dermatology*. 2nd ed. Oxford University Press. © Oxford University Press 2016. Reproduced with permission of the licensor via PLSClear.

Q1.   What is the most common causative organism for the aforementioned condition in Fig. 11.1?
Q2.   What are the main risk factors for developing this condition?
Q3.   What is the treatment?

Answers

A1.

Staphylococcus aureus is the most common, while some streptococcal and Gram-negative organisms can be causative alongside herpes simplex.

A2.

Risk factors for paronychia include acute injury to the nail folds, occupational injury to the nail folds (irritant exposure, for example), cuticle cutting, and ingrown nail.

A3.

Treatment includes saline nail soaks, and incision and drainage if there is frank pus. If there is no improvement or spreading cellulitis, then systemic antibiotics are indicated.

Further Reading

BMJ. Paronychia. 2015. Available from: http://bestpractice.bmj.com/best-practice/monograph/350.html

SAQ 10 **Retained Foreign Body**

A 42-year-old carpenter attends the emergency department, claiming that he has a retained wooden splinter in the palm of his non-dominant left hand. You can see a puncture wound but are unable to palpate any foreign body.

Q1. How would you confirm the presence and location of the splinter?
Q2. What are the immediate treatment priorities?
Q3. What is the definitive management?

Answers

A1.

Ultrasound would be a sensible start. Other imaging techniques are CT or MRI scan. Plain film radiology would not be useful.

A2.

Check on tetanus prophylaxis status and treat as indicated. Consider broad-spectrum antibiotic cover.

A3.

Referral to a hand surgeon for removal in a bloodless field in the operating theatre is indicated.

SAQ 11 Acute Respiratory Distress Syndrome

A 55-year-old patient was admitted to your resuscitation room six hours ago with pancreatitis. The intensive care unit (ICU) and medical teams have been involved from an early stage and aggressive fluid therapy instituted. There are no beds on ICU at present.

You review the patient and find that there are widespread coarse crackles all over the chest. The patient has poor urine output (20 ml in the last two hours), a heart rate of 105 bpm, and blood pressure of 110/90 mm Hg.

You request an arterial blood gas (on 15 litres oxygen per minute) which shows:

pH   7.28 PaO_2 12.40 $PaCO_2$ 6.61 FiO_2 0.8

You request a chest X-ray (see Fig. 11.2).

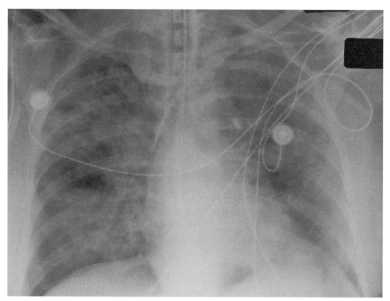

Fig. 11.2 Reproduced from Webb, A., Angus, D., Finfer, S., Gattinoni, L. and Singer, M. (2016). *Oxford Textbook of Critical Care*. 2nd ed. Oxford University Press. © Oxford University Press 2016. Reproduced with permission of the licensor via PLSClear.

Q1. What is the diagnosis?

Q2. What processes brought this about?

Q3. How should the therapy be changed to improve the current situation?

Answers

A1.

The diagnosis is acute respiratory distress syndrome (ARDS).

A2.

Widespread damage to the capillary endothelium leads to extravasation of protein rich fluid and interstitial oedema. The alveolar basement membrane is damaged, and fluid seeps into the airspaces, stiffening the lungs, and causing ventilation–perfusion mismatch.

A3.

The patient is overfilled and will need inotropic/vasopressor support rather than more fluids. Continuous positive airway pressure or intubation might be required.

The principles of mechanical ventilation are simple:

- Give enough oxygen to keep the PaO_2 over 8 kPa.
- Avoid volutrauma and barotrauma, by keeping the tidal volumes in the 4–6 ml/kg range and the airway plateau pressure below 30–35 cmH_2O (the tidal volume should not be less than 4 ml/kg, irrespective of airway pressure).
- The PaO_2 is a function of the FiO_2, the positive end-expiratory pressure (PEEP) level, the mean airway pressure, and the minute ventilation. The tidal volume, depending on what mode of ventilation is used, is determined by the pressure control level (in pressure-controlled modes) or the tidal volume dialled up on the ventilator (in volume-controlled modes).
- Move to ICU setting as soon as possible for PiCCO/LiDCO/PA-pressures.
- Senior ICU involvement is essential at this stage.

Further Reading

BMJ Best Practice. *Acute Respiratory Distress Syndrome*. Available from: http://bestpractice.bmj.com/best-practice/monograph/374/treatment/step-by-step.html

SAQ 12 **Pneumonia**

A 62-year-old man presents with productive cough, fever, and shortness of breath to the emergency department. The FY2 diagnoses a community-acquired pneumonia.

Q1. What scoring tool can you use to assess the risk of mortality?
Q2. Your patient scores 0, what antibiotic does NICE recommend you discharge him with?
Q3. List four intrathoracic complications of pneumonia.

Answers

A1.

CURB 65 score.

Confusion, urea more than 7, respiratory rate over 30/minute, blood pressure less than 90 systolic/60 diastolic, and age over 65 years. Scores of 0–1 are low risk (<3% mortality rate), 2 is an intermediate risk (3–15% mortality rate) and more than 2 is high risk (>15% mortality rate).

A2.

Low-risk patients (CURB score 0–1): consider a five-day course of amoxicillin for low-risk patients and a macrolide or tetracycline if penicillin allergic. Moderate- to high-risk patients are recommended a 7–10 course of dual therapy (amoxicillin + macrolide for moderate risk, beta-lactamase stable beta-lactam, and macrolide for high risk).

(Reproduced from *Thorax*, Lim, W.S. et al. Defining community acquired pneumonia severity on presentation to hospital: an international derivation and validation study. 2003; 58:377–82. http://dx.doi.org/10.1136/thorax.58.5.377. Copyright © 2003, BMJ Publishing Group Ltd and the British Thoracic Society. With permission from BMJ Publishing Group Ltd.)

A3.

Pneumonia can be complicated by:

- Pleural effusion (a parapneumonic exudative effusion)
- Empyema
- Lung abscess
- Atelectasis
- Pericarditis

Further Reading

NICE. *Pneumonia Overview.* Available from: https://pathways.nice.org.uk/pathways/pneumonia

SAQ 13 **Meningococcal Septicaemia**

A mother brings her 11-year-old son into the emergency department with a non-blanching skin rash. He has had a fever and started vomiting this morning. You suspect meningococcal septicaemia.

Q1. What treatment (route and dose) would you start immediately?
Q2. If you suspect meningococcal septicaemia, what investigations would you initiate in the emergency department?
Q3. What differential diagnoses would you consider?

Answers

A1.

Ceftriaxone 80 mg/kg intravenous should be administered. The NICE guidelines currently state that if a child attends with a purpuric rash, start intravenous ceftriaxone (80 mg/kg IV) immediately if the rash is spreading, there are signs of bacterial meningitis or meningococcal septicaemia, or the child appears unwell to the clinician.

A2.

Start with the basic investigations of full blood count, C-reactive protein, clotting screen, blood cultures, blood gases and, if available, consider whole blood polymerase chain reaction (PCR) for *Neisseria meningitidis*.

A3.

The differential diagnoses include Henoch–Schönlein Purpura (HSP), trauma, immune thrombocytopenia (ITP), haemolytic uraemic syndrome (HUS), and thrombotic thrombocytopenia purpura (TTP) in adults.

   HSP occurs between the ages of 3 to 15 and is characterized by:

* Palpable purpura without thrombocytopenia/clotting abnormalities
* Arthritis/arthralgia
* Gastrointestinal symptoms: abdominal pain, nausea
* Haematuria/proteinuria

Further Reading

Meningitis Research Foundation. Available at: http://www.meningitis.org/health-professionals/hospital-protocols-paediatrics

SAQ 14 **Acute Tonsillitis**

A 4-year-old child is brought in with a two-day history of cough and fever up to 38.7°C. His throat is red and you do not feel any anterior cervical lymphadenopathy.

Q1. What scoring system can you use to predict the likelihood of bacterial infection?
Q2. What are the criteria of this score?
Q3. How does the final score affect your management?

Answers

A1.

Centor score can be used to predict bacterial infection.

A2.

- One point for fever over 38.3°C
- One point for tonsillar exudate
- One point for tender anterior cervical lymphadenopathy
- One point for presence of cough

Data from Centor RM; Witherspoon JM; Dalton HP; Brody CE; Link K (1981). "The diagnosis of strep throat in adults in the emergency room". *Medical Decision Making*. 1 (3): 239–246. doi:10.1177/0272989x8100100304. PMID 6763125.

A3.

A Centor score of 3–4 has a positive predictive value of 40–60% for positive bacterial throat swabs: a course of antibiotics is recommended. A score less than 3 has a negative predictive value of 80%.

Further Reading

BMJ Best Practice. *Acute Tonsillitis*. Available from: http://bestpractice.bmj.com/best-practice/monograph/598/diagnosis/criteria.html

SAQ 15 **Tetanus Prophylaxis**

A 27-year-old farm labourer attends hospital with an incised wound to the palm of the right hand, which is contaminated with soil. You are concerned about the risk of tetanus.

Q1. List four features indicating a tetanus-prone wound.
Q2. What is the indication for human tetanus immunoglobulin?
Q3. List four clinical features of tetanus.

Answers

A1.

Tetanus-prone wounds can be recognized by the following:

- A wound or burn with a greater than six-hour delay to surgical intervention
- A wound that:
  - Is of puncture type
  - Contains a significant degree of devitalized tissue, such as a crush injury
  - Is contaminated with soil or manure
  - Contains a foreign body
  - Is infected
- Burns

A2.

Human tetanus immunoglobulin is indicated in the presence of a tetanus-prone wound and one of the two following situations:

- Last of three-dose course or reinforcing dose given 10 or more years previously: HATI + reinforcing dose of adsorbed vaccine (given at different sites)
- Not immunised or uncertain immunisation status: HATI + full three-dose course of adsorbed vaccine (given at different sites)

The dose is 250 IU intramuscular, or 500 IU if more than 24 hours since injury or there is a risk of heavy contamination or following burns.

A3.

The symptoms of generalized tetanus can be summarized by ROAST: rigidity, opisthotonus, autonomic dysfunction (sympathetic overactivity), spasms, and trismus (masseteric spasm). Other forms of tetanus include cephalic (involving cranial nerve musculature) and local (localized rigidity and spasms in the area close to the site of injury).

Further Reading

Public Health England. *Tetanus: Information for Health Professionals*. 2018. Available from: https://assets.publishing. service.gov.uk/government/uploads/system/uploads/attachment_data/file/754976/Tetanus_information_ for_health_professionals.pdf

SAQ 16 **Necrotizing Fasciitis**

A 32-year-old male attends the emergency department with severe pain, redness, and swelling of the right leg, high fever, and inability to bear weight. He has already been commenced on oral antibiotics for a diagnosis of cellulitis by his general practitioner two days previously, but his condition continues to progress. On examination, he appears toxic. On local examination, there is widespread induration extending beyond the redness on his lower leg, and a few haemorrhagic bullae in the involved skin.

Q1. What is the likely diagnosis?
Q2. What are the clinical types of this condition?
Q3. What are the principles of management? List three.

Answers

A1.

Necrotizing fasciitis is the most likely diagnosis. It must be considered in any patient with a cellulitis-like presentation associated with systemic toxicity, severe and worsening pain that appears out of proportion to the extent of skin involvement, purple or mottled skin discolouration and blister formation, induration, palpable crepitus, and 'dish-water' fluid discharge.

A2.

There are two main types, which differ according to causative organism and clinical presentation:

- Type 1 (polymicrobial synergistic infection caused by various species of Gram-positive cocci, Gram-negative bacilli, and anaerobes)
- Type 2 (monomicrobial, usually group A β-haemolytic streptococcal infection)

A3.

Management includes:

- Fluid resuscitation and haemodynamic support
- Intravenous broad-spectrum antibiotics
- Surgical referral with a view to early radical debridement

There is no proven benefit from hyperbaric oxygen therapy.

Further Reading

Hakkarainen TW, Kopari NM, Pham TN, Evans HL. Necrotizing soft tissue infections: review and current concepts in treatment, systems of care, and outcomes. *Current Problems in Surgery*. 2014;51:344–62.

Chapter 12 **Maxillofacial Surgery**

SAQ 1 **Fractured Mandible**

It is Saturday evening, and a 35-year-old man is next to be seen, He is in a minors' area cubicle. The triage note says 'Facial injury? Jaw fracture'. He has had a radiograph (see Fig. 12.1).

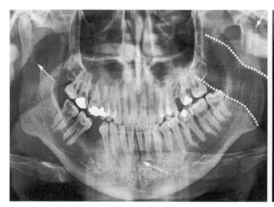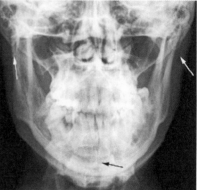

Fig. 12.1 Reproduced from *Emergency Medicine Journal*, Ceallaigh PÓ, Ekanaykaee K, Beirne CJ, et al., Diagnosis and management of common maxillofacial injuries in the emergency department. Part 2: mandibular fractures, 23, pp. 927-928. http://dx.doi.org/10.1136/emj.2006.035956. Copyright © 2006, BMJ Publishing Group Ltd and the British Association for Accident and Emergencey Medicine. With permission from the BMJ Publishing Group Ltd.

Q1. The radiograph shows multiple fractures of the mandible. Which is more common, fractures involving the condylar process, or those not involving the condylar process?

Q2. Give four features which need to be examined for when assessing a suspected mandibular fracture.

Q3. How may the airway be affected by a mandibular fracture?

Answers

A1.

Non-condylar fractures are more common, accounting for 65–75% of mandibular fractures. Road traffic accidents are more commonly associated with condylar fractures, whereas assaults more frequently lead to fractures of the angle of the mandible.

A2.

Any four of:

- Look for any gingival tear
- Look for stepping of or displaced teeth
- Feel for mobility within the mandible itself
- Look for sublingual haematoma, which though this is not sensitive for, is very specific

- Ask the patient if tooth-bite feels normal (checking for normal occlusion)
- Feel for crepitus inside and outside the mouth
- Feel for tenderness inside and outside the mouth
- Check for loose/missing teeth or broken dentures (consider chest radiograph for possibly inhaled fragments)
- Feel for tenderness at the temporomandibular joint
- Look for bleeding or haematoma in the external auditory meatus (associated with condylar neck fracture)
- Look for grazed chin plus trismus (associated with condylar fracture)

A3.

Airway compromise may be associated with mandibular fracture as a result of:

- A flail mandible associated with bilateral anterior mandibular fracture (parasymphyseal or body) causing loss of support of tongue muscles with posterior displacement of the base of the tongue. Manual anterior distraction of the mandible may be required to maintain airway patency.
- Oral bleeding and sublingual haematoma can cause airway obstruction.

Further Reading

Ceallaigh PO, Ekanaykaee K, Beirne CJ, Patton DW. Diagnosis and management of common maxillofacial injuries in the emergency department. Part 2: mandibular fractures. *Emergency Medicine Journal.* 2006;23 (10):927–8.

Nasser M, Pandis N, Fleming PS, Fedorowicz Z, Ellis E, Ali K. Interventions for the management of mandibular fractures. *Cochrane Database of Systematic Reviews.* 2013;7:CD006087.

SAQ 2 **Orbital Fracture**

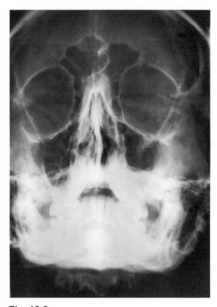

Fig. 12.2

Q1. List two abnormalities on the X-ray in Fig. 12.2.

Q2. What is the diagnosis?

Q3. What specific nerve injury must you consider, and what would be the examination findings in that instance?

Answers

A1.

The X-ray shows infraorbital irregularity, a fluid level within the maxillary sinus, and a tear drop sign caused by herniation of periorbital fat through the infraorbital rim, all on the left side.

A2.

The diagnosis is fracture of the left orbital floor.

A3.

After a fracture of the floor of the orbit, the infraorbital nerve may become trapped, producing an area of anaesthesia in the cheek, upper lip, lateral aspect of the nose, and the maxillary incisor teeth and associated gingiva.

Further Reading

Boyette JR, Pemberton JD, Bonilla-Velez J. Management of orbital fractures: challenges and solutions. *Clinical Ophthalmology*. 2015;9:2127–37.

SAQ 3 **Parotid Trauma**

A 32-year-old man presents to the department following an assault. He has multiple cuts and bruises to his limbs and lots of facial bruising and swelling with a laceration to the left side of his face. He has no evidence of chest or abdominal trauma and is haemodynamically stable.

Q1. His amylase comes back at four times the upper limit of normal—what is the likely explanation?
Q2. If this explanation is suspected how might significant injury be simply diagnosed clinically in this patient?
Q3. Is imaging likely to be beneficial?

Answers

A1.

In view of no evidence of abdominal trauma (although occult trauma remains possible) the more likely diagnosis would be traumatic parotitis secondary to blunt trauma and/or direct laceration to the parotid.

A2.

By palpating the gland, saliva may then pool in the wound demonstrating damage to the duct. Another option would be to cannulate the parotid duct and inject diluted methylene blue dye into the duct to see if there is any pooling in the wound.

A3.

Usually computed tomography (CT)/MR scan is not very useful and parotid trauma is better diagnosed clinically. Sialography may have a place but is more applicable to chronic duct obstruction.

Further Reading

Lazaridou M, Iliopoulos C, Antoniades K, Tilaveridis I, Dimitrakopoulos I, Lazaridis N. Salivary gland trauma: a review of diagnosis and treatment. *Craniomaxillofacial Trauma and Reconstruction*. 2012;5(4):189–96.

SAQ 4 **Facial Fractures**

Q1. What are the clinical features of a maxilla fracture? List three.

Q2. What is considered as the gold standard imaging for the assessment of a mandibular injury?

Q3. Which neurological structures may be compromised by a mandibular fracture?

Answers

A1.

The clinical features of maxillary fracture include:

- Malocclusion
- Surgical emphysema in the cheek
- Facial asymmetry
- Infraorbital paraesthesia
- Trismus
- Mobility of maxillary teeth
- Widening of the palate
- Bruising in the soft palate

A2.

Orthopantomogram, which provides a panoramic image of the mandible, is considered as the gold standard for routine imaging of mandibular injuries. CT scanning may occasionally be required for further characterization of condylar region injuries.

A3.

Mandibular fractures can be complicated by injury to the inferior alveolar nerve in the inferior dental canal or mental foramen, leading to numbness over the point of the chin.

Further Reading

Deangelis, AF, Barrowman, RA, Harrod, R et al. Maxillofacial emergencies: Dentoalveolar and temporomandibular joint trauma. Emergency Medicine Australasia, 2014, 26: 439-445

SAQ 5 **Avulsed Tooth**

A 28-year-old lady presents frantically to the emergency department reception. She has fallen and avulsed her upper left incisor. She has brought her tooth with her, wrapped in tissue paper. There is currently a delay of three hours to see a maxillofacial surgeon.

Q1. If the injury occurred in the last 20 minutes, what do you tell her about the chances of a successful reimplantation?

Q2. What are the primary goals of reimplantation?

Q3. List three potential contraindications for reimplantation.

Answers

A1.

An avulsed tooth should ideally be replaced within 30 minutes; this offers an over 90% chance of success if the tooth has been stored and handled appropriately. The tooth should be stored in normal saline or milk pending reimplantation. Ideally, immediate reimplantation following irrigation of the tooth socket for clot removal is preferable, pending splintage.

A2.

Early reimplantation allows for:

- Restoration of dental occlusion
- Maximization of the lifespan of the reimplanted tooth

A3.

Potential contraindications for reimplantation include:

- Poorly controlled epileptics—potential of displacement and inhalation during a seizure
- Severe learning difficulties
- Cardiac defects with a risk of infective endocarditis—a dead tooth is a potential source of infection
- Immunosuppression
- Poor compliance with treatment/poor dentition

Further Reading

Deangelis, AF, Barrowman, RA, Harrod, R et al. Maxillofacial emergencies: Dentoalveolar and temporomandibular joint trauma. Emergency Medicine Australasia, 2014, 26: 439-445

Chapter 13 **Metabolic Conditions**

SAQ 1 **Hypercalcaemia**

A 78-year-old man with known skeletal metastases from bronchial carcinoma attends the department with nausea, abdominal pain, confusion, and lethargy. You suspect hypercalcaemia, which is confirmed, with a corrected serum calcium level of 3.54 mmol/L.

Q1. What change on the electrocardiogram (ECG) are you most likely to see associated with this man's hypercalcaemia?

Q2. What single therapeutic intervention should be initiated in the emergency department?

Q3. Aside from his underlying neoplasm, name one medication that might be contributing to this man's high calcium.

Answers

A1.

A shortened QT interval, secondary to shortening or absence of the ST segment, is the commonest change on the ECG with hypercalcaemia. Other features such as a widening, flattening, inversion, or notching of T waves, or J-point elevation mimicking ST segment elevation myocardial infarction are possible, though less common. J waves may be seen with severe hypercalcaemia (3.75–4.0 mmol/L).

A2.

Intravenous rehydration with 0.9% normal saline. Nephrogenic diabetes insipidus develops due to the hypercalcaemia, leading to dehydration, which is compounded by nausea, vomiting, and lethargy, further reducing intake. If rehydration does not normalize the levels, consider adding 40 mg furosemide or a bisphosphonate (30 mg IV pamidronate, for example).

A3.

Any of the following medications may contribute to hypercalcaemia:

- Thiazide diuretics
- Lithium
- Vitamin D
- Vitamin A
- Calcium coprescribed with antacids or calcium and vitamin D preparations ('calcium-alkali syndrome')

Nearly 90% of cases of hypercalcaemia are caused by primary hyperparathyroidism or malignancy. Other causes include medication use, immobility with Paget's disease, or sarcoidosis. The symptoms can be remembered by 'moans, groans, stones and bones:

- Moans: depression, lethargy
- Abdominal groans: constipation, nausea, vomiting, and pancreatitis
- Renal stones
- Bones: osteitis fibrosa cystica, osteomalacia

Further Reading

Ahmed R, Hashiba K. Reliability of QT intervals as indicators of clinical hypercalcemia. *Clinical Cardiology*. 1988;11:395–400.

Minisola S, Pepe J, Piemonte S, Cipriani C. The diagnosis and management of hypercalcaemia. *British Medical Journal*. 2015;350:h2723.

NICE. *Hypercalcaemia—NICE CKS*. 2014. Available from: http://cks.nice.org.uk/hypercalcaemia

SAQ 2 Hypokalaemia

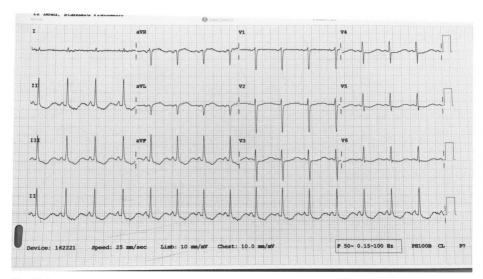

Fig. 13.1

Q1.   Which electrolyte disturbance should be suspected given this ECG in Fig. 13.1?

Q2.   What symptoms/signs might be expected in this patient? List three.

Q3.   Which other electrolyte needs to be checked as depletion is often associated with hypokalaemia?

Answers

A1.

The ECG suggests hypokalaemia. A potassium level less than 2.7 mmol/L can produce a widened taller P wave, a prolonged PR interval, T wave flattening (the earliest change) and inversion, ST segment depression, pseudo-prolongation of the QT interval (a QU interval with an absent T wave), and prominent U waves (a positive deflection after the T wave). As time goes on and potassium reduces further, more life-threatening arrhythmias may develop ranging from supraventricular tachyarrhythmias to ventricular tachyarrhythmias, including torsades de pointes and ventricular fibrillation.

A2.

Lethargy and muscle cramps might be expected in this patient. Symptoms or signs may not be reported but could include weakness, constipation, cramps, respiratory problems, palpitations, and even ascending paralysis

A3.

Magnesium may need to be replaced. Magnesium is often lost along potassium from the gastrointestinal tract or due to diuretic therapy. If low, it should be replaced as this will allow quicker potassium correction.

Further Reading

Barrett KE, Boitano S, Barman SM, Brooks HL. *Ganong's Review of Medical Physiology*. 24th edition. New York: McGraw Hill Lange; 2012.

Cohn J, Kowey P, Whelton P, Prisant M. New guidelines for potassium replacement in clinical practice. *Archives of Internal Medicine*. 2000 Sep 11;160(16):2429–36.

SAQ 3 **Acute Kidney Injury**

Marjorie, a 44-year-old lady, comes to the emergency department with diarrhoea and vomiting, feeling generally unwell and lethargic. She has type I diabetes mellitus, hypertension, and is on painkillers for a recently diagnosed left renal stone on her last visit to the ED 10 days ago.

On being shown an ECG the FY2 thought she had tall T waves, performed a venous blood gas analysis, and asks for your help:

pH 7.18	pCO_2 3.5	pO_2 8.7	HCO_3 8	BE-12	
Na 145	K8.7	Ur 42.3	ion Ca 1.56	glucose 5.6	Hb 12.5

Q1. What diagnosis do you suspect given this venous gas? Give three possible reasons for Marjorie's presentation.

Q2. Outline the management priority in this case, excluding ABC.

Q3. On treating Marjorie, she develops tetany. Why is this? How would you treat it?

Answers

A1.

Acute kidney injury (not likely chronic as her haemoglobin is normal). Possible causes include:

- Dehydration from diarrhoea and vomiting
- Diabetic ketoacidosis as she is diabetic and has a metabolic acidosis
- ACE inhibitor therapy (as hypertensive)
- Non-steroidal anti-inflammatory drugs (NSAIDs) for analgesia with renal colic
- Contrast nephropathy after renal colic investigation

A2.

Urgent treatment of hyperkalaemia involves administration of 10 units soluble insulin intravenously, followed by a bolus of 50 ml of 50% glucose, to shift the potassium into the cells. Use 10 ml of 10% calcium chloride for cardioprotection and nebulized salbutamol. Consider sodium bicarbonate and, in failure of treatment already outlined, haemodialysis.

Further management points are:

- Intravenous access and blood tests including full blood count, urea and electrolytes, glucose, coagulation screen, liver function tests, and blood cultures
- Arterial blood gases to exclude hypoxaemia (fluid overload)
- Central access and monitoring of central venous pressure to guide fluid replacement
- In view of acidosis and high potassium, 100 ml of 8.4% sodium bicarbonate intravenously
- Urine dipstick testing and microscopy plus hourly output
- Chest X-ray
- Consider ultrasound scan if no obvious cause for acute kidney injury is identified.

A3.

She developed hypocalcaemia: give further calcium if needed. Correction of acidaemia causes ionized calcium to fall. Treat with intravenous calcium or, if mild, oral calcium carbonate.

Further Reading

NICE. *Acute Kidney Injury: Prevention, Detection and Management CG169.* 2017. Available at: https://www.nice.org.
   uk/guidance/conditions-and-diseases/kidney-conditions/acute-kidney-injury

SAQ 4 **Acute Kidney Injury 2**

Errol is a 75-year-old man with known prostate cancer who attends with malaise, nausea, and confusion for 48 hours. He has recently been taking diclofenac from his general practitioner for a 'bad back'. He is seen by your FY2 who has the following results but is not sure what they mean.

Na 144   K 5.8   Ur 14   Cr 220   CCa 2.89

Q1.   What abnormalities are present and what diagnosis does this suggest?

Q2.   What immediate investigations would you request (list four)?

Q3.   A urinary catheter is inserted which yields a residual of 1400 ml. How would this alter your differential diagnosis?

Answers

A1.

Hyperkalaemia, raised urea and creatinine, hypercalcaemia. These are suggestive of acute kidney injury. Consider malignancy.

A2.

Any of the following investigations:

- Full blood count
- Clotting screen
- Urine culture
- Urinary electrolytes
- 12-lead ECG
- Chest X-ray
- Lumbar spine X-ray
- Ultrasound scan of the renal tract

A3.

In addition to acute tubular necrosis from NSAIDs, an obstructive cause is also possible. He may also have a prerenal element from dehydration, but this is impossible to assess from the information given.

Further Reading

London AKI Network. Available from: https://www.thinkkidneys.nhs.uk/aki/education/london-aki-network-academy/

SAQ 5 **Anion Gap**

Q1. Describe how the anion gap is calculated, and state the normal range.

Q2. What constitutes the majority of unmeasured anions?

Q3. List five causes of a raised anion gap.

Answers

A1.

The anion gap is calculated by subtracting the predominant measured anions from the predominant measured cations:

Anion gap = (Sodium + Potassium)—(Chloride + Bicarbonate). The overall charge is neutral and thus the anion gap is reflective of anions that are not accounted for in laboratory measurements. A raised anion gap suggests the presence of exogenous acid (e.g. ketones, poisons, lactate). The exogenous acid is buffered by, and accordingly causes a drop in the bicarbonate level, and this leads to a raised anion gap. The normal range is 8–16 mmol/L.

A2.

Albumin comprises most unmeasured anions.

A3.

Any of the following (the mnemonic is MUDPILES):

M—Methanol

U—Uraemia

D—Diabetic ketoacidosis/alcoholic ketoacidosis

P—Paraldehyde/phenformin

I—Iron/isoniazid

L—Lactic acidosis

E—Ethylene glycol

S—Salicylates

Further Reading

Kraut JA, Nagami GT. The serum anion gap in the evaluation of acid-base disorders: what are its limitations and can its effectiveness be improved? *Clinical Journal of the American Society of Nephrology*: CJASN. 2013;(8)11:2018–24.

SAQ 6 **Exercise-induced Hyponatraemia**

A 25-year-old female has been running a half-marathon. She has collapsed during the course of the race and has been brought to the hospital for further assessment, as she remains drowsy. In the emergency department she is afebrile and blood tests are done. The venous blood gas shows pH 7.35, Na 116, K 3.6, HCO3 21, lactate 3.2

Q1. What is the likely diagnosis?
Q2. What are the mechanisms by which this condition can arise? List two.
Q3. What specific treatment would you recommend?

Answers

A1.

Exercise-induced hyponatraemia.

A2.

The mechanism of production can be multifactorial, including:

- Dilutional, with a fluid intake greater than body fluid losses during first 24 hours after exercise. Fluids that are hypotonic or pure water will exacerbate the dilutional effect. Isotonic liquids are recommended.
- Sodium loss through excessive sweating.
- Inappropriate antidiuretic hormone (ADH) release in exercise.

Risk factors that have been mentioned include:

- Female sex (this may be related to a lower body mass index)
- Long distance athletic event, lasting more than 4 hours (endurance events: marathons; ultra-marathons; triathlons)
- More than 3 litres of fluid ingested
- Weight gain during race
- Low body mass index
- Slow race pace

A3.

Hypertonic saline, as she has severe hyponatraemia and continued drowsiness. Give 100 ml 3% saline intravenous boluses; repeat up to three times at 10-minute intervals if required. Administration in small boluses is safe, with no reports of adverse consequences of treatment. Restoration of a normal level of consciousness is the end-point of treatment. No hypotonic or isotonic solutions should be administered.

Treatment of hyponatraemia depends on the severity of the patient's symptoms:

- Mild to moderate (alert and oriented): salty snacks/broths; no oral fluids until onset of urination
- Severe, with neurological complications: hypertonic saline

Further Reading

Hew-Butler T, Loi V, Pani A, Rosner MH. Exercise-associated hyponatremia: 2017 update. *Frontiers in Medicine*. 2017;4:21.

SAQ 7 **Severe Hyponatraemia**

A 65-year-old female is brought to the resuscitation room following a generalized tonic-clonic seizure. On arrival, she is drowsy, with a Glasgow Coma Score of 13/15. Her vital signs are: heart rate 84/minute, respiratory rate 18/minute, blood pressure 110/80 mm Hg. A venous blood gas is obtained, which shows the following: Na 115; K 3.7; HCO3 22; creatinine 75.

Q1. How would you interpret the blood findings?
Q2. What specific treatment should be considered?
Q3. What are the potential risks of rapid treatment?

Answers

A1.

This patient has severe hyponatraemia.
  The causes of hyponatraemia can be broadly categorized as follows:

- Renal losses (urinary Na >20 mmol/L; patient dry; causes are Addison's, renal failure, diuretics)
- Extrarenal losses (urinary Na <20 mmol/L; patient dry; burns, vomiting, diarrhoea, small bowel obstruction, fistulae)
- Organ failures (patient overloaded; nephrotic syndrome, heart failure, liver failure, renal failure)
- SIADH (patient is euvolaemic with high urinary osmolality; always consider malignancy)

A2.

In the presence of likely neurological complications (such as headache, confusion, drowsiness, and seizures), intravenous hypertonic (3%) saline should be administered, 100 ml intravenous bolus over 10 to 15 minutes, with ongoing monitoring of serum sodium. The aim of treatment is to raise serum sodium by 4–6 mmol/L.

A3.

Inappropriately rapid correction may result in brain dehydration, central pontine myelinolysis, cerebral haemorrhage, or congestive heart failure.

Further Reading

Verbalis JG, Goldsmith SR, Greenberg A, Korzelius C, Schrier RW, Sterns RH, et al. Diagnosis, evaluation, and treatment of hyponatraemia: expert panel recommendations. *American Journal of Medicine*. 2013;126:510–42.

Chapter 14 **Musculoskeletal Conditions**

SAQ 1 **Septic Arthritis**

A 62-year-old woman presents to your department with a three-day history of a swollen and painful left knee. There is no history of trauma. She has no past medical history and her observations are normal. Her knee is swollen and feels warm.

Q1. You worry she might suffer from septic arthritis of her knee. How would you confirm the diagnosis?

Q2. Give two risk factors for septic arthritis.

Q3. What bacteria are most frequently involved? List two.

Answers

A1.

The diagnosis of septic arthritis can be confirmed by synovial aspiration. All patients with a short history of hot, red, and swollen joints should be considered having septic arthritis until proven otherwise. The best way to diagnose septic arthritis is to perform a synovial fluid aspiration. The septic joint aspirate is often opaque, has a yellow to greenish colour, high white cell count, and is often positive on culture.

NB: It is interesting to note that the British Society of Rheumatologists state that neither the absence of organisms on Gram stain nor a negative synovial fluid culture excludes the diagnosis of septic arthritis.

A2.

Any of the following are risk factors for septic arthritis:

- Old age (>80 years)
- Immunosuppression
- Pre-existing arthritis: rheumatoid arthritis; osteoarthritis
- Intravenous drug user
- Prosthetic joint
- Intra-articular injection
- Cellulitis; cutaneous ulcers
- Diabetes mellitus

A3.

The most common causative agent is *Staphylococcus aureus*.

Streptococci and Gram-negative bacilli have also been found to be causative organisms. *Neisseria gonorrhoeae* is the most common cause in young, sexually active adults.

Further Reading

BMJ Best Practice. *Septic Arthritis*. Available from: http://bestpractice.bmj.com/best-practice/monograph/486/treatment/guidelines.html

Coakley G, Mathews C, Field M, Jones A, Kingsley G, Walker D, et al. BSR & BHPR, BOA, RCGP and BSAC guidelines for management of the hot swollen joint in adults. *Rheumatology*. 2006;45:1039–41.

SAQ 2 **Buckle Fracture**

A 4-year-old girl comes in to the department having fallen onto her outstretched hand. She is quite tender over her wrist, however, there is no swelling. An X-ray is performed; see Fig. 14.1.

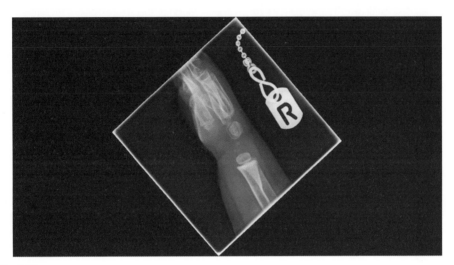

Fig. 14.1

Q1. What is the diagnosis?
Q2. What is the preferred management strategy for immobilization?
Q3. What is the preferred follow-up strategy?

Answers

A1.
She has a minimally displaced buckle fracture of the distal radius.

A buckle fracture, often referred to as *torus* fracture, is a very common injury pattern in children. Children have softer more flexible bones and thus, following an injury, there is often an angulation of the cortex on *one* side, as though it has buckled.

A2.
Three weeks' use of a Futura splint (or less if child is comfortable). A cast may be considered if pain relief is not effective enough in the splint.

A3.

No follow-up is usually required.

The splint can be safely removed by the parents. If there is pain, a return to the emergency department is recommended. The child should avoid contact sport for 6 weeks.

Further Reading

RCEM. *Distal Forearm Buckle Fractures in Children*. Available from: https://www.rcem.ac.uk/docs/Local%20 Guidelines_Paediatric/12d.%20Distal%20Forearm%20Buckle%20Fractures%20in%20Children%20 (Addenbrooke's%20Hospital,%202009).doc

SAQ 3 **Scaphoid Fracture**

A 20-year-old male falls onto his outstretched left hand and presents to your emergency department with wrist pain. The experienced triage nurse sends him for a wrist X-ray, which is shown in Fig. 14.2.

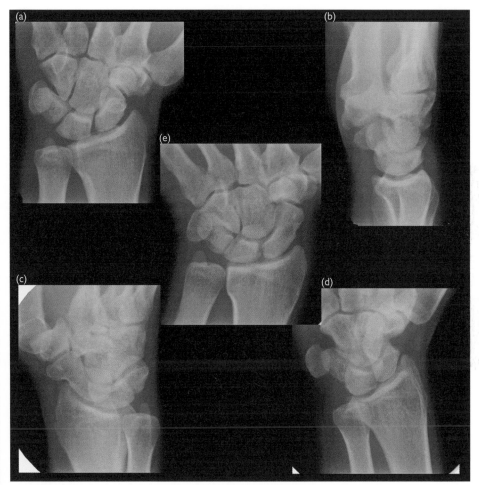

Fig. 14.2 Reproduced with permission from Bulstrode, C. et al. (2011). *Oxford Textbook of Trauma and Orthopaedics*. 2nd ed. Oxford University Press. © Oxford University Press 2011. Reproduced with permission of the licensor via PLSClear.

Q1. What is the diagnosis and what are the likely clinical examination findings?

Q2. What are the tendons that form the borders of the anatomical snuffbox?

Q3. If a repeat X-ray one week later is negative but suspicion of a scaphoid fracture remains, what further investigation would you suggest?

Answers

A1.

The diagnosis is a scaphoid fracture. Notice the subtle cortical disruption through the waist of the scaphoid on the radial side.

Examination findings are:

- Anatomical snuffbox tenderness
- Scaphoid tubercle tenderness
- Pain on telescoping the thumb into the scaphoid

A2.

The anatomical snuffbox has the following boundaries:

- Medial border: extensor pollicis longus
- Lateral border: extensor pollicis brevis and abductor pollicis longus

A3.

Magnetic resonance imaging will confirm or rule out the diagnosis.

Further Reading

RCEM. *Guideline for the Management of Suspected Scaphoid Fractures in the Emergency Department.* Available from: https://www.rcem.ac.uk/docs/College%20Guidelines/5z25.%20Suspected%20Scaphoid%20Fractures-%20(Flowchart)%20(Sept%202013).pdf

SAQ 4 **Kohler's Disease**

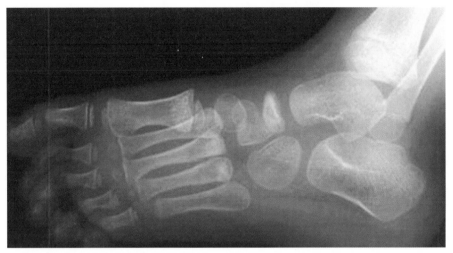

Fig. 14.3 Reproduced with permission from Bulstrode, C. et al. (2011). *Oxford Textbook of Trauma and Orthopaedics*. 2nd ed. Oxford University Press. © Oxford University Press 2011. Reproduced with permission of the licensor via PLSClear.

Q1. What is the abnormality on the X-ray in Fig. 14.3)?

Q2. What is the cause of this radiological appearance?

Q3. Name two other bones that can undergo a similar condition and the eponymous name used to describe them.

Answers

A1.

Osteochondrosis of the navicular bone, also known as Kohler's disease. This is characterized by sclerosis, collapse, and fragmentation of the involved bone. The X-ray shows a sclerotic ossific nucleus.

A2.

Temporary loss of blood supply causes aseptic ischaemic necrosis of the bone. The condition is self-limiting, and typically affects epiphyseal ossification centres.

A3.

Any of the following are examples of osteochondrosis:

- Kienböck's disease—lunate
- Perthes' disease—femoral head
- Panner's disease—humeral capitellum
- Sinding–Larsen disease—inferior pole of patella
- Osgood–Schlatter disease—tibial tubercle
- Sever's disease—calcaneal apophysis
- Freiberg's disease—metatarsal head
- Scheuermann's disease—anterior vertebral end-plates

SAQ 5 **Dislocated Ankle**

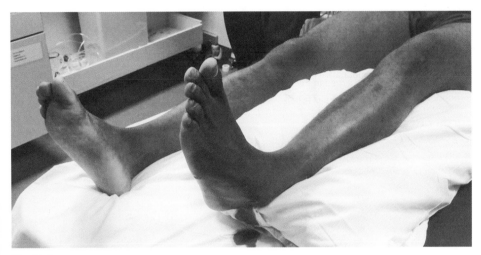

Fig. 14.4

Q1. Please see Fig. 14.4. You are asked to prioritize this patient. What are the patient implications of delaying treatment?

Q2. You decide to use procedural sedation. List three patient features that may affect airway management.

Q3. List three criteria that must be satisfied before a patient is discharged after procedural sedation.

Answers

A1.

The crucial point in that an ankle fracture dislocation (whether open or closed) is a limb-threatening condition, owing to vascular compromise, and therefore requires immediate reduction in order to restore anatomical alignment. Other complications of delaying treatment are skin and soft tissue devitalization, pressure sores, and unrelieved pain.

A2.

Any of the following may affect airway management (list three):

- Dysmorphic or asymmetrical facial features
- A beard
- Significant malnutrition or cachexia with sunken cheeks and missing teeth

- Facial trauma, particularly lacerations through the cheek or unstable bony injuries
- Limited neck extension
- Obesity
- Poor mouth opening of less than 4–5 cm which restricts access

A3.

All of the following should be fulfilled prior to discharge home:

- The patient is alert and orientated.
- Vital signs are stable and within acceptable limits.
- Patients should be discharged in the presence of a responsible adult who will accompany them home and be able to report any post-procedure complications.

Further Reading

RCEM. *Pharmacological Agents for Procedural Sedation and Analgesia in the Emergency.* 2017. Available from: http://www.rcem.ac.uk/docs/College%20Guidelines/Pharmacological%20Agents%20for%20Procedural%20Sedation%20and%20Analgesia%20(Jan%202017%20Revised).pdf

SAQ 6 **Humeral Fracture**

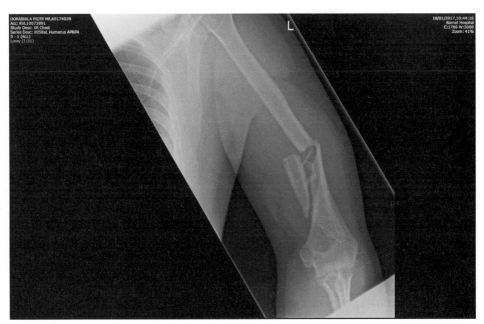

Fig. 14.5

Fig. 14.5 is a plain radiograph of a 32-year-old male brought in after falling off a moped, presenting with pain and swelling in the left arm.

Q1. Describe the image in Fig. 14.5.

Q2. What neurological structure may have been injured? If so, what might you find on neurological examination?

Q3. What are the indications for surgical fixation of humeral fractures? List two.

Answers

A1.

The plain anteroposterior radiograph of the left humerus shows an angulated, displaced, and comminuted fracture of the middle third of the humerus.

A2.

The radial nerve might be injured, usually as a neuropraxia caused by stretching or shearing, but occasionally is entrapped in the fracture or lacerated. The radial nerve runs along the spiral groove in the mid-humerus. Injury to the radial nerve may manifest as:

- Wrist drop
- Weakness of supination of the forearm
- Loss of extension of the fingers
- Sensory deficit involves the skin overlying the first dorsal interosseous space

A3.

Indications for operative fixation of the humerus include:

- Unacceptable position following reduction
- In the context of polytrauma (two or more distinct anatomical regions injured)
- Open humeral fractures
- Segmental humeral fractures
- Pathological fractures

Further Reading

BMJ Best Practice. *General Long Bone Fracture Management Guidelines.* Available from: http://bestpractice.bmj.com/best-practice/monograph/386/treatment/step-by-step.html

SAQ 7 **Ankle Fractures**

The next patient in the triage queue has a 'painful, swollen ankle following a fall'.

Q1.   What are the Ottawa ankle rules for deciding whether an X-ray is required?
Q2.   What is a Maisonneuve fracture?
Q3.   In what circumstances can an isolated lateral malleolar fracture be managed non-operatively?

Answers

A1.

The Ottawa ankle rules indicate plain X-rays of the ankle following trauma in the presence of:

- Point tenderness at the posterior edge of the distal 6 cm or tip of the lateral malleolus
- Point tenderness at the posterior edge of the distal 6 cm or tip of the medial malleolus
- Inability to bear weight for four steps immediately after the injury and in the emergency department

A2.

This is an eponymously named fracture complex consisting of:

- High fibular fracture
- Separation of the tibiofibular syndesmosis
- Fracture of the medial malleolus OR rupture of the medial ankle ligament complex—this is usually caused by pronation with external rotation and is an unstable fracture requiring surgery

A3.

An isolated lateral malleolar fracture can be managed conservatively if:

- The fracture is undisplaced or minimally displaced
- There is congruent mortise
- There is no talar shift

Management in a short-leg cast for 6 weeks is acceptable with weight-bearing for the final 3 weeks. Any talar shift will require either 6 weeks in a non-weight-bearing cast OR open reduction with internal fixation (this becomes the only option if any displacement is non-reducible).

Further Reading

BMJ. *Ankle Fractures*. 2016. Available from: http://bestpractice.bmj.com/best-practice/monograph-pdf/385.pdf

SAQ 8 **Rotator Cuff Injury**

A 63-year-old man has been exercising his dog in the park and presents with a painful shoulder following a particularly vigorous throw of a ball. You suspect a rotator cuff injury.

Q1.   What is the 'empty-can' test and what injury is it testing for?
Q2.   What two other injuries you will test for if you suspect rotator cuff injury?
Q3.   Which rotator cuff muscle is not usually tested for and why?

Answers

A1.

The empty-can test is a test for a tear of the supraspinatus.

Both arms should be raised slightly forward from the trunk's coronal plane, both thumbs pointing to the floor (as if emptying a can). To test for weakness of the supraspinatus, pressure must be applied to the top of the arms and the patient should actively resist.

A2.

You will test for infraspinatus and subscapularis injuries:

- Test for infraspinatus tears (by getting the patient to hold their elbows tight to their side, elbows flexed at 90 degrees, they must then externally rotate against resistance).
- Test for injury to the subscapularis muscle by performing the 'lift-off', test which assesses the ability of the patient to lift a hand away from the small of their back against resistance.
- An alternative is the 'belly-press test' in which the patient presses their hand against their own umbilicus with the elbow held to the side. Resistance is tested by an examiner attempting to lift the patients hand away from their abdomen.

A3.

Specific testing for teres minor tends not to be performed as it essentially performs the same action as the infraspinatus (external rotation), although at certain positions it has more impact—such as when the arm is above the head pushing upward as if protecting oneself from a falling object from above.

Further Reading

BMJ Best Practice. *Rotator Cuff Injury*. 2016. Available from: http://bestpractice.bmj.com/best-practice/monograph-pdf/586.pdf

SAQ 9 **Elbow Dislocation**

A 40-year-old male is seen in the emergency department after radiographic examination of his left elbow following trauma. It reveals a posterior dislocation of the elbow with no associated fracture.

Q1.   What are the key examination findings to document in this patient and how will you examine for them? List four.
Q2.   What is the management in this case?
Q3.   What are the components of the terrible triad of elbow injuries?

Answers

A1.

Document the function of radial, ulnar, and median nerves.

   Function of the radial (thumb, finger, and wrist extension and dorsal hand sensation), ulnar (finger abduction and ulnar border of hand sensation), and median (finger flexion and palmar and thenar eminence sensation) nerves, as well as patency of the brachial artery (via equal bilateral radial pulses) must be documented before any attempt at reduction.

A2.

The elbow needs to be relocated under, ideally, procedural sedation. Initially the elbow should be extended to 30 degrees of flexion. The overall alignment of the elbow then needs to be restored by centring the olecranon between the medial and lateral epicondyles. With longitudinal traction applied to the forearm, and countertraction to the humerus, the elbow is flexed slowly to 90 degrees. Further flexion of the elbow and direct downward pressure to the olecranon should result in a 'clunk' as the joint reduces. Prior to repeat radiograph, the elbow should be splinted at 90 degrees of flexion with neutral forearm rotation. Neurovascular examination is paramount once the patient has recovered adequately from sedation.

A3.

The terrible triad (so-named as there is little to maintain stability of the elbow) of injuries comprise:

- Dislocation of the elbow
- Fracture of the coronoid process of the ulna
- Fracture of the radial head

This combination of injuries requires ORIF (open reduction and internal fixation).

Further Reading

BMJ. *Joint Dislocation*. 2016. Available from: http://bestpractice.bmj.com/best-practice/monograph-pdf/583.pdf

SAQ 10 **Occult Hip Fracture**

You have examined an 85-year-old female who is unable to bear weight on the left leg following a fall. She has severe pain in the left groin, associated with local tenderness. Plain X-rays of the pelvis and left hip do not reveal an obvious fracture. You wonder whether she might have sustained an occult hip fracture

Q1.   What are the features suggestive of an occult hip fracture?
Q2.   What options can be considered for investigation?
Q3.   What might be the consequences of failure of diagnosis?

Answers

A1.

The triad of inability to straight leg raise, groin tenderness, and painful limitation of hip rotation may indicate the diagnosis.

Axial loading of the leg (telescoping the femur into the acetabulum) may produce hip pain.

A2.

MRI scan is recommended by NICE.

Computed tomography (CT) scan is suggested as a diagnostic option if MRI is not available within 24 hours or is contraindicated.

Admission and repeat hip X-ray may allow delineation of the fracture line by bone resorption along the fracture line, impaction, or displacement.

Radionuclide bone scan.

A3.

Displacement at the fracture site
Avascular necrosis of the femoral head
Thromboembolism

Further Reading

NICE. *Hip Fracture: Management CG124.* 2017. Available from: https://www.nice.org.uk/guidance/cg124
Rajkumar S, Tay S. Clinical triad for diagnosing occult hip fractures with normal radiographs. *Journal of Orthopaedic Surgery.* 2005;3:1–3.

SAQ 11 **Back Pain**

A Foundation Year 2 (FY2) in the emergency department asks for your help to assess a 48-year-old builder with acute back pain of spontaneous onset.

Q1. List four red flag signs and/or symptoms of back pain.
Q2. Fill Table 14.1 with the names of the deep tendon reflex nerve roots.
Q3. Describe Brown–Sequard syndrome.

Table 14.1

Biceps

Triceps

Supinator

Knee

Ankle

Answers

A1.

Any of the following are red flag symptoms or signs of back pain:

- Thoracic pain
- Bowel/bladder incontinence/retention
- Saddle anaesthesia
- Reduced anal tone
- Neurological deficit
- Bilateral radiculopathy

A2.

The deep tendon reflex nerve roots are listed in Table 14.2.

Table 14.2

Biceps	C5 C6
Triceps	C7 C8
Supinator	C5 C6
Knee	L3 L4
Ankle	S1

A3.

The abnormal neurology in Brown–Sequard syndrome is as follows:

- Ipsilateral—motor paralysis and loss of proprioception and vibration (corticospinal tracts and dorsal columns)
- Contralateral—loss of temperature and pain (spinothalamic tracts, which decussate)

Further Reading

NICE. *Low Back Pain CG88*. 2009. Available from: https://www.nice.org.uk/guidance/cg88

NICE. *Selection of Patients for CT Head and CT Cervical Spine CG56*. Available from: https://www.nice.org.uk/guidance/cg176/resources/imaging-algorithm-pdf-498950893

SAQ 12 **Chest Injury**

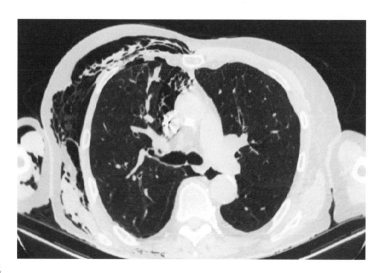

Fig. 14.6

Q1. List three abnormalities on the scan in Fig. 14.6).

Q2. What are the landmarks for a surgical chest drain?

Q3. What sedative agent could you use to supplement the local anaesthetic?

Answers

A1.

The CT scan in Fig. 14.6 shows:

- Pneumothorax
- Rib fracture
- Surgical emphysema

A2.

The anatomical landmarks for chest drain placement are: between fourth/fifth intercostal space in the anterior axillary line (i.e. within the triangle of safety: anterior to latissimus dorsi and posterior to lateral border of pectoralis major, and above fifth intercostal space).

A3.

Ketamine or morphine are useful adjuncts.

Further Reading

Trauma.org. *Chest Trauma: Intercostal Chest Drains.* Available from: http://www.trauma.org/archive/thoracic/CHESTdrain.html

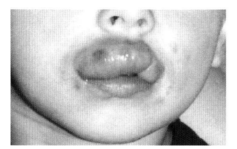

Fig. 5.2 Figure 21.4 from 'Urticarial rashes', p0, *Paediatric Dermatology* (Oxford Specialist Handbook of Paediatrics) by Sue Lewis Jones Copyright (2010) Oxford University Press.

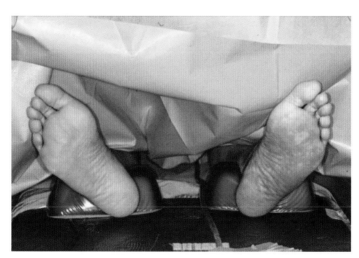

Fig. 6.1 Image A of fig. 4.1.2 from Chapter 4.1 'Acute Lower Limb Ischaemia', p0, in *Oxford Textbook of Vascular Surgery* by Matthew M. Thompson et al, Robert Fitridge, Jon Boyle, Matt Thompson, Karim Brohi, Robert J. Hinchliffe, Nick Cheshire, A. Ross Naylor, Ian Loftus, and Alun H. Davies. Copyright (2016) Oxford University Press.

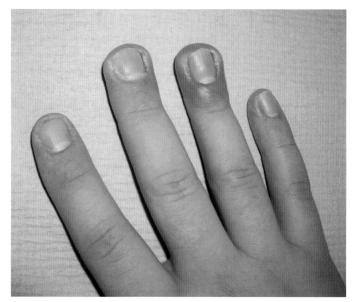

Fig. 11.1 Fig 18. 5 from Chapter 18 'Cutaneous reactions to drugs', p0, in *The Oxford Handbook of Medical Dermatology* edited by Susan Burge, Rubeta Matin, and Dinny Wallis. Copyright (2016) Oxford University Press.

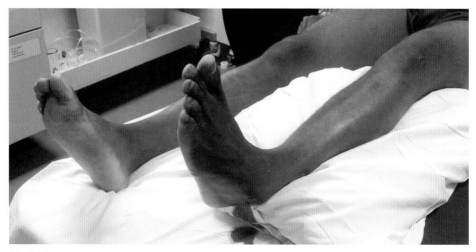

Fig. 14.4

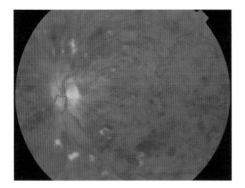

Fig. 17.2 Reproduced from Fig 6.27, Chapter 6, p0, *Training in Ophthalmology* (2nd edition), edited by Venki Sundaram, Allon Barsam, Lucy Barker, and Peng Tee Khaw. Copyright (2016) Oxford University Press.

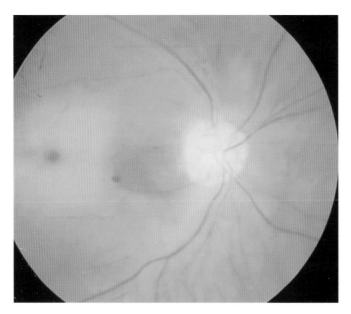

Fig. 17.3 Reproduced from Fig 6.27, Chapter 6, p0, *Training in Ophthalmology* (2nd edition), edited by Venki Sundaram, Allon Barsam, Lucy Barker, and Peng Tee Khaw. Copyright (2016) Oxford University Press.

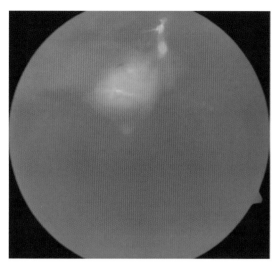

Fig. 17.4 Reproduced from Fig 5.17, p0, *Training in Ophthalmology* (2nd edition), edited by Venki Sundaram, Allon Barsam, Lucy Barker, and Peng Tee Khaw. Copyright (2016) Oxford University Press.

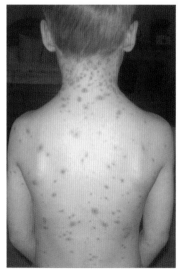

Fig. 18.3 Reproduced from Fig. 25.3 in Chapter 25, p0, *Paediatric Dermatology* (Oxford Specialist Handbooks in Paediatrics), edited by Sue Lewis-Jones. Copyright (2010) Oxford University Press.

SAQ 13 **Perilunate Dislocation**

A 45-year-old-male presents following a fall off a motorcycle with wrist pain and swelling. Figs. 14.7a and b show a lateral X-ray of his wrist.

(a)

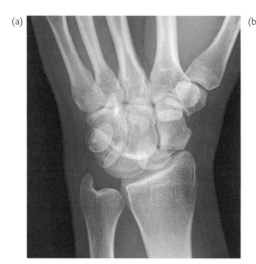

(b)

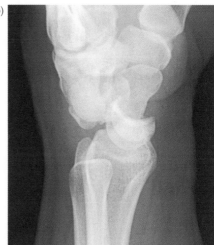

Fig. 14.7

(a) Reproduced with permission from Anderson, M. and Smith, S. (2013). *Musculoskeletal Imaging Cases.* Oxford University Press USA. © Oxford University Press 2014. Reproduced with permission of the licensor via PLSClear.

(b) Reproduced with permission from Anderson, M. and Smith, S. (2013). *Musculoskeletal Imaging Cases.* Oxford University Press USA. © Oxford University Press 2014. Reproduced with permission of the licensor via PLSClear.

Q1. Describe the abnormality seen in Figs. 14.7a and b.

Q2. What is the likely mechanism?

Q3. What is the likely prognosis of this injury?

Answers

A1.

Figs. 14.7a and b show a lateral X-ray of the left wrist revealing a perilunate dislocation of the carpus. The lunate remains in anatomical position with respect to the distal radius, and the entire carpus dislocates dorsally relative to it. The capitate no longer articulates with the lunate, which presents with an empty cup distally.

In a lunate dislocation, the lunate bone dislocates anteriorly and its concave surface then faces volarly or anteriorly, giving the 'spilled teacup' appearance.

These injuries can be overlooked radiologically, especially with lack of awareness of the radiological patterns.

A2.

The mechanism of injury is a fall onto the outstretched hand, involving high-energy impact.

A3.

Most cases develop post-traumatic arthritis, though there is evidence that early ORIF may reduce the risk. Other acceptable answers include median nerve dysfunction, complex regional pain syndrome, and carpal instability.

Further Reading

Navaratnam Annakan V, Ball S, Emerson C, Eckersley R. Perilunate dislocation. *BMJ*. 2012;345:e7026.

SAQ 14 **Pulled Elbow**

A two-year-old girl is brought to the emergency department. She is refusing to use the left upper limb, which is held fully extended at the elbow with the forearm pronated. It is noted that she has been playing with her older brother, aged nine. There is no history of any specific documented injury

Q1. What is the likely diagnosis?
Q2. What is the pathogenesis of this condition?
Q3. Describe the management.

Answers

A1.

The likely diagnosis is a pulled elbow or nursemaid's elbow.

A2.

Pulled elbow is associated with radial head subluxation, which is commonest in children aged one to four years. The radial head subluxes from the annular ligament, which is interposed in the radiocapitellar joint.

A3.

Manipulation is recommended. Relocation is often achieved by supination of the forearm, along with flexion of the elbow while maintaining pressure on the radial head. A click may be felt. Usually the child commences use of the upper limb within 5–10 minutes.

Further Reading

OrthoInfo. *Nursemaid's Elbow*. Available at: http://orthoinfo.aaos.org/topic.cfm?topic=a00717

SAQ 15 **Sternal Fracture**

A young male patient presents to the department following blunt chest trauma. He has sustained an undisplaced sternal fracture.

Q1. What other injuries should be sought evidence of in this patient? List three.
Q2. He has no other injuries and is asymptomatic. Should cardiac biomarkers be measured?
Q3. What do you need to warn this man about?

Answers

A1.

Common accompanying injuries include:

- Cervical spine fractures
- Multiple rib fractures
- Thoracic vertebral fractures
- Lung contusions (usually when rib fractures also present)
- Myocardial contusion
- Aortic injury

A2.

No. With an isolated, undisplaced sternal fracture there is no good evidence for measuring biomarkers of cardiac injury. A normal 12-lead electrocardiogram (ECG) is reassuring. In patients with no cardiac concerns (such as history of cardiac disease, arrhythmias, haemodynamic instability) it is unlikely that cardiac investigations will be abnormal in an asymptomatic patient with suspected myocardial contusion. If cardiac biomarkers are raised, this is usually a benign finding (not predictive of further cardiac complications) and no treatment is required.

A3.

Very often these patients have long-standing pain associated with their injury and therefore adequate analgesia will be required once discharged.

Further Reading

Hossain M, Ramavath A, Kulangara J, Andrew JG. Current management of isolated sternal fractures in the UK: time for evidence-based practice? A cross-sectional survey and review of literature. *Injury*. 2010;41(5):495–8.

Chapter 15 **Neurology and Psychiatry**

SAQ 1 **Herpes Zoster Ophthalmicus**

A 72-year-old woman presents with a vesicular rash over the left side of her forehead and around her left eye. She describes feeling unwell prior to appearance of the vesicles and complains of significant pain in the area of the rash. You suspect this lady has developed shingles in the distribution of the ophthalmic branch of the trigeminal nerve. You take a more detailed history and examine her.

Q1. As a part of your assessment, you examine for Hutchinson's sign. What is this?
Q2. Is herpes zoster ophthalmicus (HZO) contagious?
Q3. Who should be treated with antiviral medications when presenting with HZO?

Answers

A1.

Hutchinson's sign describes the appearance of herpes zoster lesions in the distribution of the nasociliary dermatome (inner corner of the eye, side of the nose, and tip of the nose) and this is a prognostic sign for further ocular involvement. See Fig. 15.1.

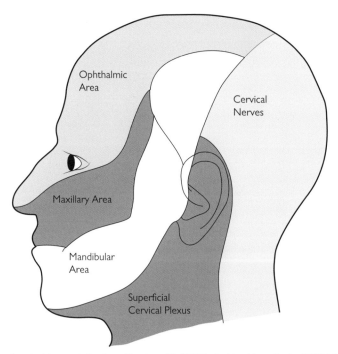

Fig. 15.1 Reproduced with permission from Harrison, M. (2017). *Revision Notes for the FRCEM Primary*. 2nd ed. Oxford University Press. © Oxford University Press 2017. Reproduced with permission of the licensor via PLSClear.

A2.

If a person who has never been exposed to varicella-zoster virus (i.e. with chickenpox) comes into contact with someone suffering with HZO, before all the vesicles crust over, then they are at risk of developing chickenpox. In other words, herpes zoster is contagious in the active vesicular stage.

A3.

Anyone presenting with herpes zoster in the ophthalmic distribution of the trigeminal nerve should receive antiviral therapy, aciclovir 800 mg orally five times daily for seven days, ideally commenced within 72 hours. In immunocompromised individuals, aciclovir treatment should be continued for two days after crusting of the lesions. This reduces the duration and severity of symptoms and reduces the risk of complications, particularly post-herpetic neuralgia.

Further Reading

Ting DSJ, Ghosh N, Ghosh S. Herpes zoster ophthalmicus. *BMJ*. 2019;364:k5234.

SAQ 2 **Stroke**

A 62-year-old man presents with a history of left-sided facial weakness and slurred speech which lasted 15 minutes and has now completely resolved. Examination reveals a heart rate of about 90 beats per minute, which is irregular, a blood pressure of 120/85 mm Hg and a normal neurological examination. He has no past medical history of note. While in the emergency department (ED), he becomes increasingly unresponsive and is found to have left-sided facial weakness, confused speech, and a left-sided hemiparesis.

Q1. Define what is meant by a stroke.
Q2. What is the Rosier score and what is this patient's score?
Q3. List four contraindications for stroke thrombolysis.

Answers

A1.

Stroke refers to acute focal or global neurological deficit, of vascular origin, lasting more than 24 hours or leading to death, and including cerebral infarction, intracerebral haemorrhage, and subarachnoid haemorrhage. Hypoglycaemia should be excluded as a cause of symptoms. Urgent brain imaging is essential to exclude intracerebral haemorrhage and stroke mimics (such as subdural haematoma and intracranial space-occupying lesions), particularly if stroke thrombolysis with alteplase is contemplated. In practice, the 24-hour limit which forms part of the World Health Organization (WHO) definition of stroke is becoming obsolete, as anyone with ongoing neurological deficit within the 24-hour time frame should be treated as having had a stroke. While the definition of transient ischaemic attack allows for resolution within 24 hours, most resolve within an hour.

A2.

'Recognition of Stroke in the Emergency Room' is a scoring system recommended by National Institute for Health and Care Excellence (NICE) to aid clinicians in the diagnosis of stroke in the ED.

One point is given for any of the following: asymmetrical arm leg weakness; asymmetrical leg weakness; asymmetrical facial weakness; speech disturbance; and visual field defect. One point is subtracted for any of the following: seizure, loss of consciousness. If zero or less, a stroke is unlikely. This patient's score is 2.

A3.

Contraindications for stroke thrombolysis include:

- Haemorrhagic stroke or haemorrhagic transformation of ischaemic stroke (on computed tomography (CT) head scan)
- Known bleeding diathesis
- Major surgery within last 14 days
- Severe head injury and/or neurosurgery within last 3 months

- History of brain tumour, intracranial arteriovenous malformation, or aneurysm
- Seizure at stroke onset
- Active internal bleeding

Further Reading

Minhas JS, Robinson TG. Latest developments in clinical stroke care *Journal of the Royal College of Physicians of Edinburgh*. 2017;47:360–3.

NICE. *Stroke and Transient Ischaemic Attack in Over 16s: Diagnosis and Initial Management CG68*. 2017. Available from: https://www.nice.org.uk/guidance/cg68

Nor AM, Davis J, Sen B, Shipsey D, Louw SJ, Dyker AG, et al. The Recognition of Stroke in the Emergency Room (ROSIER) scale: development and validation of a stroke recognition instrument, *The Lancet Neurology*. 2005;4:727–34.

SAQ 3 **Transient Ischaemic Attack**

A 75-year-old male presents following an hour-long episode of dysphasia and right-sided upper and lower limb weakness, which has now resolved. He has a past medical history of hypertension, type 2 diabetes mellitus, and hyperlipidaemia. His vital signs are: heart rate 80 per minute, blood pressure 150/100 mm Hg, respiratory rate 18, and oxygen saturation on room air of 95%.

Q1. What is his ABCD2 score?
Q2. What anatomical territory is likely to be involved?
Q3. What investigations should be considered?

Answers

A1.

His ABCD2 score is 7

- Age: >= 60 years: 1 point
- Blood pressure >= 140/90 mm Hg: 1 point
- Clinical features:
  Unilateral weakness: 2 points
  Speech disturbance without weakness: 1 point
- Duration: >= 60 minutes: 2 points; 10–59 minutes: 1 point
- Presence of diabetes mellitus: 1 point

Data from Perry, J.J. et al. Prospective validation of the ABCD2 score for patients in the emergency department with transient ischaemic attack. *Canadian Medical Association Journal*, 2011, 183 (10): 1137-1145. https://doi.org/10.1503/cmaj.101668.
High risk of stroke is associated with a Rosier score ≥ 4.

A2.

The middle cerebral artery territory is likely to be involved.
The basilar and internal carotid arteries form the Circle of Willis, at the base of the brain, from which the three major supplying cerebral arteries emerge:

- Anterior cerebral artery (infarction of this territory produces a weak numb contralateral leg. Arm symptoms are milder, and the face is spared. Bilateral infarction produces akinetic mutism).
- Middle cerebral artery (the most commonly affected territory in a stroke; infarction may produce contralateral hemiparesis of mainly the face and arm and contralateral homonymous hemianopia, and dysphasia if the dominant hemisphere is affected).
- Posterior cerebral artery (infarction may produce contralateral homonymous hemianopia or quadratic visual field defects, cortical blindness, crossed syndromes of ipsilateral cranial nerve palsy and contralateral long motor or sensory tract dysfunction, or diplopia, vertigo, ataxia, dysarthria, and dysphagia). Recognition of ischaemia in the posterior cerebral artery can be difficult, as the presentation can be non-specific and not relate to a FAST-positive situation.

A3.

Investigations to be undertaken, or considered, in a patient presenting with a stroke and depending on individual circumstances, include:

- Blood: full blood count, urea and electrolytes, glucose, cholesterol, and triglycerides, erythrocyte sedimentation rate, syphilis serology
- Arteries: carotid and vertebral artery Doppler ultrasound
- Heart: 12-lead electrocardiogram (ECG), echocardiography
- Brain imaging: CT and/or MRI scan

Further Reading

Gommans J, Barber AP, Fink J. Preventing strokes: the assessment and management of people with transient ischaemic attack. *N Z Med J*. 2009;122(1293);3556.

Perry JJ, Sharma M, Sivilotti ML, Sutherland J, Symington C, Worster A, et al. Prospective validation of the ABCD2 score for patients in the emergency department with transient ischaemic attack. *Canadian Medical Association Journal*. 2011;183:1137–45.

SAQ 4 **Ventriculo-peritoneal Shunt Complications**

A 23-year-old female with a history of cerebral palsy is brought in by the ambulance after a seizure lasting two minutes. She has a ventriculo-peritoneal shunt *in situ*. Her mother tells you she had been vomiting all morning.

Q1. Other than vomiting and seizures, what other symptoms would indicate a blocked ventriculo-peritoneal shunt?

Q2. What investigations would you perform in the emergency department to evaluate the shunt?

Q3. She starts fitting. For her initial management, what is the pharmacological agent of choice?

Answers

A1.

Drowsiness, headache, optic disc swelling with or without visual symptoms and occasional failure of upward gaze are all signs of possible ventriculo-peritoneal shunt blockage. Atypical presentations include abdominal mass due to pseudocyst (a loculated fluid collection), cranial nerve palsies, and hemiparesis. Early recognition of the possibility of shunt blockage is essential to prevent major neurological complications, including blindness, and death. Presenting symptoms are often non-specific.

A2.

Specific investigations to evaluate shunt function in the emergency setting include a CT head scan to look for evidence of hydrocephalus and a shunt series of X-rays (of skull, chest, and abdomen) to track the shunt itself to detect any obvious causes of discontinuity in the catheter, such as fracture, disconnection, migration, or malposition.

A3.

Administration of 4 mg intravenous lorazepam is the first-line treatment for a seizure. The seizure management algorithm suggests a maximum of two initial doses of benzodiazepine (by whichever route of administration) followed by a loading dose of phenytoin (20 mg/kg) if fitting continues.

Further Reading

Paff M, Alexandru-Abrams D, Muhonen M, Loudon W. Ventriculoperitoneal shunt complications: a review. *Interdisciplinary Neurosurgery*. 2018;13:66–70.

SAQ 5 **Seizures**

A 25-year-old known epileptic is brought directly to the resuscitation room with an ongoing general-ized tonic-clonic seizure, the onset of which was around 20 minutes previously. He has received 10 mg rectal diazepam prior to arriving in hospital.

Q1. List some likely precipitants for his seizure.
Q2. Summarize the fitting patient algorithm.
Q3. List four potential complications of this condition.

Answers

A1.

Precipitants for status epilepticus include:

- Antiepileptic drug withdrawal
- Central nervous system infections
- Alcohol intoxication or withdrawal
- Traumatic brain injury
- Metabolic disturbance
- Recreational drug use (e.g. sympathomimetic agents)
- New medication (e.g. antipsychotic drugs)

A2.

The protocol for management of an ongoing seizure includes:

Airway, Breathing, Circulation, Disability, Exposure (ABCD) protocol
Early intravenous access
Rapid seizure termination with antiepileptic medication

a) Lorazepam 0.05–0.10 mg/kg intravenous bolus over 2 minutes (maximum 4 mg). A further single dose can be given after 10 minutes. Thus, up to two initial doses of benzodiazepine are recommended. Diazepam, 0.3 mg/kg intravenous over 2 minutes (maximum 10 mg), is an alternative. Repeated doses may be required as diazepam is rapidly redistributed (high volume of distribution owing to high lipid solubility).
b) Loading dose of phenytoin, 20 mg/kg IV over 20 minutes, diluted in normal saline (rate not exceeding 50 mg per minute), with continuous ECG monitoring. Alternatively give phenobarbital 10–20 mg/kg IV (maximum rate:100 mg/minute), followed by maintenance dose of 1–4 mg/kg/day.
c) Rapid sequence induction with propofol, midazolam, or thiopental sodium and suxamethonium, followed by rapid placement of an endotracheal tube.

In addition, intravenous glucose (50 ml of 50% solution) and/or thiamine (250 mg), and Pabrinex® are recommended if there is any suggestion of alcohol abuse or impaired nutritional status.

A3.

Complications of status epilepticus include:

- Airway-related complications, including obstruction or aspiration
- Respiratory acidosis
- Cardiac arrhythmias
- Rhabdomyolysis; acute kidney injury
- Neurogenic pulmonary oedema
- Hyperthermia
- Disseminated intravascular coagulation
- Skeletal trauma (spinal fracture, posterior shoulder dislocation)

Further Reading

NICE. *Epilepsies: Diagnosis and Management CG137.* 2018. Available from: https://www.nice.org.uk/guidance/cg137

SAQ 6 **Alcoholism/Wernicke's Encephalopathy**

A 45-year-old male with a history of alcohol abuse is brought to the emergency department drowsy and confused following a witnessed generalized seizure. There is no documented history of injury.

Q1.   What important differential diagnoses would you consider?
Q2.   List some investigations which would be useful in the initial assessment of this patient?
Q3.   List three clinical features of Wernicke's encephalopathy.

Answers

A1.

Potential causes of seizure in this patient include:

• Alcohol withdrawal or intoxication
• Hypoglycaemia
• Electrolyte disturbance
• Unrecognized traumatic brain injury (subdural haematoma)
• Central nervous system infections

A2.

Initial investigations that would be useful in establishing the cause of his symptoms include:

• Capillary blood glucose (hypoglycaemia)
• Metabolic screen (hyponatraemia/hypercalcaemia, hypocalcaemia/hypercalcaemia, hypomagnesaemia; acute kidney injury)
• Venous blood gases (lactate; rapid screen of electrolyte status)
• CT head scan/MRI scan (the latter is preferred for identification of structural abnormalities following a first seizure)

A3.

Wernicke's encephalopathy is characterized by the triad of:

• Confusion
• Cerebellar dysfunction, with gait ataxia
• Ophthalmoplegia

A useful mnemonic to aid the clinician recall the features of Wernicke-Korsakoff syndrome is 'COAT RACK':

C—Confusion

O—Ophthalmoplegia

A—Ataxia

T—Thiamine deficiency

R—Retrograde amnesia

A—Anterograde amnesia

C—Confabulation

K—Korsakoff psychosis

SAQ 7 **Wernicke's Encephalopathy 2**

One of the department's regular attenders arrives by ambulance. He has presented frequently in the past with illness or injury related to excessive alcohol consumption.

Q1.   Define Wernicke's encephalopathy.
Q2.   List three other risk factors for Wernicke's encephalopathy, besides alcohol dependence.
Q3.   What treatment should you start in the emergency department?

Answers

A1.

Wernicke's encephalopathy is an acute neuropsychiatric syndrome characterized by a potentially reversible triad of ataxia, ophthalmoplegia, and confusion due to thiamine deficiency. Thiamine depletion must be considered in alcoholics presenting with acute neuropsychiatric disturbance and treated on clinical suspicion, as the encephalopathy is reversible, and failure to treat can lead to death or permanent brain damage involving severe short-term memory loss and confabulation (Korsakoff's psychosis). This is important, as the clinical features can be misattributed to alcohol intoxication.

A2.

Risk factors for Wernicke's encephalopathy include:

- Malnutrition
- Eating disorder
- Malignancy
- HIV infection (AIDS)
- Hyperemesis

A3.

Slow intravenous administration of vitamins B and C formulated as Pabrinex®, which contains water-soluble vitamins B_1 (thiamine), B_2 (riboflavin), B_3 (nicotinamide), B_6 (pyridoxine), and C (ascorbic acid) is indicated in the emergency department. Two pairs of ampoules (1 and 2) in 100 ml saline or 5% glucose are administered over 30 minutes in the emergency department and continued during the hospital admission.

Further Reading

Galvin R, Brathen G, Ivashyna A, Hillbom M, Tanasescu R, Leone MA, et al. EFNS guidelines for the diagnosis, therapy and prevention of Wernicke encephalopathy *European Journal of Neurology*. 2010;17:1408–18.

SAQ 8 **Acute Psychosis**

A 32-year-old male, with no known past medical or psychiatric history, is brought to the hospital by the police. He is hearing threatening voices and is aggressive, and his mother phoned 999 as she was unable to cope with him. It appears that he has been demonstrating mood disturbance and has become more withdrawn over the past ten days. Initial physical examination does not reveal any sign of injury or other abnormality, and a capillary blood glucose and baseline venous blood gas analysis are within normal limits.

Q1. What is the most likely diagnosis?
Q2. What features suggest an organic cause for his presentation?
Q3. List some methods of restraining this patient as he is becoming increasingly agitated and violent.

Answers

A1.

Acute psychosis should be considered in this situation. The major symptoms of a psychotic episode are hallucinations (especially third-party auditory hallucinations), delusions (paranoid or persecutory; grandiose), confused and disturbed thought (including thought interference), and a lack of insight and self-awareness.

A2.

An organic cause for acute behavioural disorder may be suggested by:

- Recent head injury
- Recent seizures
- New onset headache
- Fluctuating level of consciousness
- Recreational drug use (e.g. sympathomimetics, cannabis)
- Fever

A3.

Restraint methods include:

- Physical restraint
- Chemical restraint (rapid tranquilization), for example, benzodiazepines (lorazepam), antipsychotic agents (haloperidol)

Further Reading

NICE. *Psychosis and Schizophrenia in Adults: Prevention and Management CG178*. 2014. Available from: https://www.nice.org.uk/guidance/cg178

SAQ 9 **Viral Encephalitis**

An 85-year-old gentleman presents with agitation, neck pain, and odd behaviour, and requires intubation and ventilation for a CT brain, which shows no acute change. The medical team suggest a lumbar puncture before any attempt is made to wake him. The cerebrospinal fluid (CSF) results are:

   WCC: 850 (80% lymphocytes); glucose: 80 mg/Dl; protein: 110 mg/dL.

Q1.   What is the likely diagnosis and what are the risk factors for it?
Q2.   What antimicrobial agent should be used for treatment?
Q3.   What further investigation(s) are needed?

Answers

A1.

The most likely diagnosis is viral encephalitis, reflected in CSF pleocytosis.

   Risk factors include extremes of age, immunodeficiency, viral illness, organ transplantation, and certain geographical locations where ticks and mosquitoes act as disease vectors.

A2.

The treatment is aciclovir intravenously 10 mg/kg three times daily, continued for 14 days. However, it is prudent to treat this patient simultaneously for bacterial meningitis in the first instance as full results are unlikely to be available immediately, involving treatment with an appropriate antibiotic such as intravenous cefotaxime PLUS amoxicillin (to cover listeriosis in this age group).

A3.

MRI scanning is the imaging of choice for diagnosis of viral encephalitis. Herpes simplex encephalitis is associated with abnormal signal and focal oedema in the temporal lobe, causing mass effect. CT scan can be normal, especially in the early stages, but may show reduced attenuation in one or both temporal lobes. Electroencephalogram (EEG) can also be useful, showing focal or generalized large slow waves.

Further Reading

Sabah M, Mulcahy J, Zeman A. Herpes simplex encephalitis. *BMJ*. 2012;344:e3166.

SAQ 10 **Subarachnoid Haemorrhage**

A 55-year-old female is brought into the resuscitation room unconscious, having suddenly collapsed while at work. As part of the diagnostic workup, a CT head scan is obtained (see Fig. 15.2).

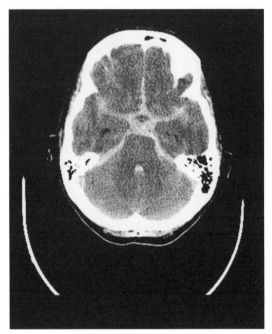

Fig. 15.2 Reproduced with permission from Cantle, F., Lacy, C. and Thenabadu, S. (2015). *Challenging Concepts in Emergency Medicine: Cases with Expert Commentary*. Oxford University Press. © Oxford University Press, 2015. Reproduced with permission of the licensor via PLSClear.

Q1. Describe the abnormality on her CT head scan as shown in Fig. 15.2.

Q2. What are your initial priorities? List three.

Q3. Describe the Glasgow Coma Scale.

Answers

A1.

The CT scan shows intracerebral and subarachnoid haemorrhage. Subarachnoid haemorrhage is characterized by the presence of hyperdense blood in the basal cisterns, Sylvian fissures, or the interhemispheric fissure, and over the convexities in the cortical sulci.

A2.

Initial management priorities include:

- Assess and secure the airway
- Blood pressure control with titrated beta-blockers (blood pressure needs to be maintained high enough to maintain cerebral perfusion pressure but not too high so as to encourage further bleeding, e.g. no higher than 130–140 mm Hg systolic)
- Arrange urgent neurosurgical consultation
- Nimodipine intravenously (1 mg/hour initially, increased after two hours in the absence of a severe fall in blood pressure)
- Agents to reduce raised intracranial pressure (mannitol, 500 ml of 20%, or hypertonic saline, 150 ml boluses of 3%), with neurosurgical advice

A3.

The Glasgow coma scale consists of (Table 15.1):

Table 15.1

		Score
Eye opening:	Spontaneous	4
	To speech	3
	To pain	2
	None	1
Verbal response:	Orientated	5
	Confused conversation	4
	Words (inappropriate)	3
	Sounds (incomprehensible)	2
	None	1
Best motor response:	Obeys commands	6
	Localizes to pain	5
	Withdrawal	4
	Flexion	3
	Extension	2
	None	1
Total coma score		3–15

Reprinted by permission from Springer-Verlag Wien: Springer Nature, Teasdale, G. et al. Adding up the Glasgow Coma Score. In: Brihaye J. et al. (eds) Proceedings of the 6th European Congress of Neurosurgery. *Acta Neurochirurgica*, vol 28. Springer, Vienna. Copyright © 1979, Springer-Verlag Wien.

Further Reading

Lawton MT, Vates GE. Subarachnoid haemorrhage. *New England Journal of Medicine*. 2017, 377: 257–66.

SAQ 11 **Thrombolysis in Stroke**

A 62-year-old male is brought to the resuscitation room after collapsing in a supermarket. On arrival, he found to have a dense right hemiplegia and is dysphasic. His Glasgow Coma Score is 14/15. His vital signs are: pulse rate 84, respiratory rate 18, and blood pressure 160/90 mm Hg. You are considering thrombolysis for a presumed acute stroke.

Q1. List four contraindications to stroke thrombolysis.

Q2. How is the severity of stroke assessed prior to thrombolysis?

Q3. What thrombolytic agent is used and in what dose?

Answers

A1.

Absolute contraindications to stroke thrombolysis include:

- History of intracranial haemorrhage, aneurysm, arteriovenous malformation, or neoplasm
- Major surgery in preceding two weeks
- Active gastrointestinal or urinary tract bleeding within previous three weeks
- Serious head injury or stroke within previous three weeks
- Coagulation disorder; anticoagulant therapy
- Extensive middle cerebral artery territory infarction on CT scan as shown by extent of hypodensity
- Severe uncontrolled hypertension: systolic blood pressure >185 mm Hg, diastolic blood pressure >110 mm Hg

A2.

The NIH Stroke Severity Score (NIHSS) is an 11-item scoring system that quantifies the degree of impairment caused by a stroke. A score of less than 5 excludes patients from tPA treatment in some centres.

A3.

Recombinant tissue plasminogen activator (rtPA or alteplase) 0.9 mg/kg to a maximum of 90 mg; 10% is given as an intravenous bolus, followed by an infusion of the remainder over 60 minutes.

Further Reading

Royal College of Physicians; Intercollegiate Stroke Working Party. *National Clinical Guideline for Stroke*, 5th edition. 2016. Available at: https://www.rcplondon.ac.uk/guidelines-policy/stroke-guidelines

SAQ 12 **First Fit**

A 25-year-old male is brought to the emergency department following a first generalized tonic-clonic seizure. He is now alert and orientated.

Q1. List three initial investigations in the emergency department.

Q2. What advice should be given on discharge home?

Q3. What are the indications for neuroimaging while in the emergency department?

Answers

A1.

Initial investigations in a person presenting following a first seizure include:

- Serum glucose
- Blood biochemistry: electrolytes, calcium, magnesium
- Venous blood gases
- 12-lead ECG

Serum prolactin is not recommended for diagnosing epilepsy.

A2.

Verbal and written advice should be given on discharge, with documentation in the emergency department records: not to drive or use machinery. They should also take sensible precautions when performing activities such as swimming or bathing until further notice. Drivers should be to advised contact the Driver and Vehicle Licensing Agency (DVLA). The employer should be informed by the patient for certain high-risk occupations (e.g. public service vehicle driver, airline pilot, and others). The patient should be advised that although he is thought to have had a seizure, this does not mean that he has epilepsy.

A3.

Neuroimaging is indicated in the presence of:

- New focal neurological deficit
- Altered mental state
- Persistent headache
- Head injury
- Malignancy
- Anticoagulation or bleeding diathesis
- Alcoholism

In the acute phase, owing to logistic reasons, this usually involves a CT head scan. MRI scanning is the imaging modality of choice for recognition of structural brain abnormalities responsible for seizures.

Further Reading

NICE. *Epilepsies: Diagnosis and Management CG137*. 2012; updated April 2018. Available from: https://www.nice.org.uk/guidance/cg137

SAQ 13 **Non-epileptic Seizures**

A 32-year-old female is brought to the emergency department following an episode of prolonged limb shaking. She continues to have several more episodes while in the ED.

Q1. What clinical features are suggestive of a non-epileptic attack disorder?
Q2. What management would you recommend?
Q3. What are the risk factors for psychogenic non-epileptic attacks? List three.

Answers

A1.

Non-epileptic attack disorder is suggested by:

- Prolonged seizure
- Vocalization in presence of bilateral motor seizures
- Situational trigger
- Bizarre movements: pelvic thrusting; bicycling leg movements
- Resisted eye opening
- Rapid recovery with no post-ictal confusion or drowsiness

A2.

The initial management includes:

- Diagnostic workup in the emergency department to exclude an organic cause, including blood tests (for electrolytes, calcium, magnesium), capillary blood glucose, venous blood gases, and CT head (in some cases), 12-lead ECG, and urine dipstick.
- Mental health referral, involving the family if possible. Psychotherapy or cognitive behavioural therapy may be indicated.

A3

Risk factors for non-epileptic attack disorder include:

- Females affected more than males
- Age of onset is late teens to early twenties
- More likely if history of childhood abuse
- Associated with personality disorders (e.g. borderline)
- Having an actual diagnosis of epilepsy can be associated with non-epileptic seizures
- History of head injury or neurosurgery

Further Reading

Perez DL, LaFrance WC, Jr. Nonepileptic seizures: an updated review. *CNS Spectrums*. 2016;21:239–46.

SAQ 14 **Mental Health Act**

A 21-year-old female attends the emergency department after an act of deliberate self-harm, having made several superficial cuts in the left forearm with a knife. The duty psychiatrist is planning to section her for a mental health assessment.

Q1. Which section of the mental health act could be used to detain the patient for assessment of the mental condition?

Q2. How many individuals should be involved in the sectioning process?

Q3. How long can the detention be applied for?

Answers

A1.

Section 2 of the Mental Health Act provides for compulsory detention in hospital for assessment, or for assessment followed by treatment, while acting in the best interests of the patient, their safety, or for the safety of others. An application for assessment requires written recommendations in the relevant form by two registered medical practitioners.

A2.

Ideally three individuals should be involved in the sectioning process: an Approved Mental Health Professional, a section 12-approved doctor, and a registered medical practitioner.

A3.

Up to 28 days of detention can be applied for. An appeal to the Mental Health Review Tribunal may be made within 14 days of admission.

Notes:

Section 2: For assessment of mental health, maximum detention time 28 days.

Section 3: For treatment of mental health (prior diagnosis/contact with services). Maximum detention up to 6 months.

Section 4: For assessment of mental health: used in emergency situations, when only one physician is available: maximum detention time 72 hours.

Section 5 relates to being able to stop patients from leaving the hospital (not ED).

Section 5.2: Doctor's holding power: maximum detention time 72 hours.

Section 5.4: Nurse's holding power: maximum detention time 6 hours.

Section 136: Authorizes a Police Officer to remove an individual, who appears to be suffering from an acute psychiatric disturbance, from a public place and transfer them to a 'place of safety' (i.e. an ED). On arrival they must be assessed psychiatrically. The section 136 lasts for up to 72 hours. If admission is required it must be converted to a Section 2 or 3. The patient under a section 136 remains under police custody throughout the period in the ED until one of the following occurs:

1. The individual is discharged from the s136 (must be undertaken by a s12 doctor or a doctor with psychiatric experience).
2. ED staff are willing to accept responsibility for the individual's custody for the purpose of mental health assessment (in which ED staff possess the legal power to detain that patient and use justifiable force if necessary).
3. The individual is conveyed to the local health-based place of safety.

Further Reading

Mental Health Act. 2007. Available from: http://www.legislation.gov.uk/search

SAQ 15 **Acute Psychosis**

A 27-year-old male is brought in by the police having been found wandering in the streets and threatening passers-by. It is possible that he is on recreational drugs. He is restless, refusing to sit still, and remains aggressive.

Q1. What are the options for management of his mental state?
Q2. What medications might be recommended for his initial treatment?
Q3. What are the requirements for safe monitoring during and after provision of this treatment?

Answers

A1.

Initial options for managing his mental state include:

- Verbal de-escalation
- Chemical restraint (rapid tranquilization)
- Seclusion and physical restraint under common law

A2.

The traditional options for rapid tranquillization include:

- Lorazepam 1–2 mg orally, intramuscularly, or intravenously (at least 30–60 minutes should be allowed between doses to allow for assessment of clinical effect)
- Haloperidol 5–10 mg intramuscularly
- Oral medication should be tried initially whenever possible

A3.

Monitoring during and after tranquillization includes:

- Continuous pulse oximetry
- ECG monitoring
- Non-invasive blood pressure and heart rate monitoring

Further Reading

Parker C. Tranquillisation of patients with aggressive or challenging behaviour. *The Pharmaceutical Journal*. 2015;294:No 7868/9.

SAQ 16 **Subarachnoid Haemorrhage**

A 35-year-old female presents with acute severe headache and neck pain. She is afebrile, with a Glasgow Coma Score of 15. There is no focal neurological deficit. You suspect subarachnoid haemorrhage (SAH).

Q1. List investigations that can be used to confirm the diagnosis.
Q2. List three risk factors for SAH.
Q3. What treatments should be considered in the ED?

Answers

A1.

SAH can be confirmed by:

- Non-contrast CT head scan (95–98% positive in first 12 hours)
- Lumbar puncture 12 hours after onset of headache if CT scan is negative for xanthochromia and bilirubin spectrophotometry
- CT angiography

A2.

Risk factors for SAH include:

- Positive family history (first-degree relatives have a five-times increased risk of a SAH)
- Hypertension
- Recreational drug use (cocaine, amphetamines)
- Excessive alcohol consumption
- Coagulopathy

A3.

Initial management includes:

- Blood pressure control to maintain systolic blood pressure below 140 mm Hg (intravenous beta-blockers or calcium channel blockers)
- Calcium channel blockers, for example, nimodipine 60 mg stat (then 6 hourly) or 1 mg/kg intravenous
- Antiemetics

Further Reading

Steiner T, Juvela S, Unterberg A, Jung C, Forsting M, Rinkel G, et al. European Stroke Organization Guidelines for the management of intracranial aneurysms and subarachnoid haemorrhage. *Cerebrovascular Diseases.* 2013;35:93–112.

SAQ 17 **Transient Ischaemic Attack 2**

A normally fit and well 65-year-old woman is brought to the emergency department with a history of speech disturbance, which lasted for 30 minutes, having occurred two days previously. She has no symptoms now. She took her blood pressure at the time with home monitor and it was 120/60 mm Hg and it remains a similar figure at present. She is not diabetic. You assess her and agree it is likely a transient ischaemic attack (TIA).

Q1. What is this lady's ABCD2 score?
Q2. Should this lady have a CT head scan?
Q3. When should this lady have imaging of her carotid arteries?

Answers

A1.

The ABCD2 score = 3:

- Age >65 scores 1
- Blood pressure >140/90—either figure for systolic or diastolic blood pressure (SBP or DBP) scores 1
- Clinical features: unilateral weakness scores 2, speech disturbance with no weakness scores 1, other symptoms score nothing
- Duration less than 10 scores nothing, 10–59 minutes scores 1, 60 minutes or more scores nothing
- Diabetes scores 0

Data from Perry, J.J. et al. Prospective validation of the ABCD2 score for patients in the emergency department with transient ischaemic attack. *Canadian Medical Association Journal*, 2011, 183 (10): 1137-1145. https://doi.org/10.1503/cmaj.101668.

A2.

Currently there is no indication for a CT scan. She will however need assessment within one week by a specialist. If she does need scanning, a diffusion-weighted magnetic resonance scan will be the modality of choice.

If she had an ABCD2 score of more than 3 or had a crescendo TIA *and* the vascular territory/pathology was uncertain, then an urgent scan would be indicated: ideally a diffusion-weighted MR scan but if not available, then a CT scan.

If her ABCD2 score was 3 or less and she did not have a crescendo TIA but if the vascular territory/pathology was uncertain, then imaging would be indicated non-urgently.

A3.

Once she has had specialist assessment, her carotid imaging should take place within one week of symptom onset because she is likely to be a candidate for endarterectomy.

There are two different cut-offs in clinical usage: 50–99% symptomatic carotid stenosis (using North American Symptomatic Carotid Endarterectomy Trial criteria) and 70–99% symptomatic carotid stenosis (using European Carotid Surgery Trialists' Collaborative Group criteria), which would indicate the need for assessment and carotid endarterectomy referral within 1 week of symptom onset. Surgery should then be performed within 2 weeks of symptom onset. Best medical treatment should also be initiated.

In those where stenosis is less than 50% or 70% (depending which criteria are adopted—this should be indicated on the scan report) surgery should not be performed, but best medical therapy should be provided (including blood pressure control, antiplatelet agents, lowering of cholesterol using medications, and diet and lifestyle advice).

Further Reading

NICE. *Stroke and Transient Ischaemic Attack in Over 16s: Diagnosis and Initial Management CG68*. 2017. Available from: https://www.nice.org.uk/guidance/cg68

Chapter 16 **Obstetrics and Gynaecology**

SAQ 1 **Advanced Life Support/Venous Thromboembolism in Pregnancy**

A 34-year-old pregnant lady attends the emergency department with left calf swelling. She is a 34/40 primipara, with no relevant past medical history. She denies any chest pain, shortness of breath, or palpitations. Your Foundation Year 2 (FY2) trainee informs you that in order to rule out deep vein thrombosis, he has sent venous blood for measurement of D-dimer and plans to discharge the patient if the blood test is negative.

Q1. According to the Royal College of Obstetricians and Gynaecologists (RCOG), what is the role of D-dimer in evaluating the pregnant patient being investigated for venous thromboembolism?

Q2. What is the best imaging modality to refute or confirm a diagnosis of lower limb deep vein thrombosis in pregnancy? How is this done?

Q3. She suddenly deteriorates and has a cardiac arrest with pulseless electrical activity. You commence cardiopulmonary resuscitation, with a few modifications for the gravid patient. Beyond what gestational age and until how long after the arrest would you initiate a peri-mortem Caesarean section?

Answers

A1.

The RCOG does not recommend testing D-dimer for the workup of venous thromboembolism (VTE) in pregnancy. There is a progressive rise in D-dimer levels throughout pregnancy, and are no agreed thresholds for a positive result.

A2.

Compression duplex ultrasound is the recommended diagnostic tool. If the scan is positive, then the patient must be treated for VTE. If the patient has a high pretest probability and if the first scan is negative then it needs to be repeated at day 3 and 7 without anticoagulant cover.

A3.

The RCOG states that if there is no response to resuscitation after four minutes, of correctly performed cardiopulmonary resuscitation (CPR), then delivery should be undertaken to assist resuscitation *if the woman is beyond 20 weeks of gestation*. This should be achieved within five minutes of cardiovascular collapse.

Ensure that the patient is in left lateral tilt beyond 20 weeks' gestation to relieve aorto-caval compression by the gravid uterus. There is emphasis to secure the airway early as pregnant women are at higher risk of regurgitation and aspiration. If a shockable rhythm is identified then use the same energy as a non-pregnant patient.

Further Reading

RCOG. *Thrombosis and Embolism During Pregnancy and the Puerperium, Reducing the Risk*. Green-Top Guideline No 37a. 2015. Available from: https://www.rcog.org.uk/en/guidelines-research-services/guidelines/gtg37a/

SAQ 2 **Pre-eclampsia**

A 34-year-old woman comes to the emergency department with her five-day-old son. Over the past three days she has developed a severe frontal headache occasionally with bright flashes in her visual field.

Q1. What is her likely diagnosis?

Q2. What bedside investigations could you perform to elucidate the diagnosis? List two.

Q3. She proceeds to have a 10 second tonic-clonic seizure in front of you. What intravenous medication would you give her to reduce the recurrence of seizures?

Answers

A1.

The likely diagnosis is pre-eclampsia. It affects 2–8% of all pregnancies and can occur from 20 weeks' gestation until a few weeks after delivery. It is defined by a new onset of hypertension and proteinuria. Severe pre-eclampsia is defined as hypertension and proteinuria with history of severe headache, visual symptoms (such as flashing lights or blurring of vision), vomiting, subcostal pain, clonus, papilloedema, liver tenderness, pulmonary oedema, thrombocytopenia, raised serum creatinine, or evidence of HELLP syndrome (haemolysis, elevated liver enzymes, and low platelet count).

A2.

Blood pressure measurements and urine dipstick analysis would confirm the likely diagnosis. The blood pressure should be greater than 140/90 mm Hg, with proteinuria 300 mg/24 hours or greater, or 1+ or greater on two random urine samples, collected at least four hours apart.

A3.

With a patient who has a seizure, load with 4 g of intravenous magnesium sulphate over 5 minutes and start an infusion of 1 g/hour over the next 24 hours. Benzodiazepines and antiepileptic drugs are not routinely recommended.

Further Reading

NICE. *Hypertension in Pregnancy: Diagnosis and Management CG107*. 2011. Available from: https://www.nice.org.uk/guidance/cg107

SAQ 3 **Pelvic Inflammatory Disease**

A 21-year-old female presents to the emergency department with lower abdominal pain and vaginal discharge.

Q1. List four causes of vaginal discharge.
Q2. List three clinical features that would suggest pelvic inflammatory disease (PID).
Q3. List two organisms involved in PID.

Answers

A1.

Possible causes of vaginal discharge include:

* Physiological discharge
* Infection or inflammation (vaginitis, cervicitis): bacterial vaginosis; sexually transmitted infections: candida albicans (vaginal thrush), trichomonas vaginalis, gonorrhoea, chlamydia, genital herpes; PID
* Foreign body (e.g. retained tampon)
* Genital tract malignancy (cervix, uterus, ovary)
* Fistulae
* Allergy

A2.

All of the following must be present for a diagnosis of PID:

* Lower abdominal pain and tenderness
* Cervical motion tenderness
* Adnexal tenderness

In addition, at least one of the following must be present:

* Oral temperature ≥38°C
* White cell count ≥10 500/cu mm
* Intrapelvic mass on examination or ultrasonography
* White blood cells and bacteria on culdocentesis (aspiration of Pouch of Douglas)
* Mucopurulent cervicitis
* ESR >15–20 mm/hour

Diagnosis of PID can be difficult, with some episodes asymptomatic or only mildly symptomatic, with non-specific symptoms. Unrecognized infections can lead to infertility. Hence a high index of suspicion must be maintained.

A3.

Possible causative organisms of PID include:

- Neisseria gonorrhoeae (aerobic)
- Chlamydia trachomatis (aerobic)
- Gardnerella vaginalis (aerobic)
- *Escherichia coli* (aerobic)
- Haemophilus influenzae (aerobic)
- Streptococcus species (aerobic)
- Bacteroides species (anaerobic)
- Peptostreptococcus species (anaerobic)
- Peptococcus species (anaerobic)
- Prevotella species (anaerobic)
- Mycoplasma species

Further Reading

British Association for Sexual Health and HIV. *UK National Guideline for the Management of Pelvic Inflammatory Disease 2011 Clinical Effectiveness Group.* 2011. Available from: https://www.bashh.org/guidelines

SAQ 4 **Ovarian Hyperstimulation Syndrome**

A 41-year-old lady presents two weeks after fertility treatment. She is short of breath, tachycardic, and complaining of lower abdominal pain and distension.

Q1. List two most likely diagnoses with this presentation.

Q2. What is the physiological mechanism of ovarian hyperstimulation syndrome?

Q3. What is the management (list three interventions)?

Answers

A1.

Differential diagnoses to consider with this presentation are:

- Ovarian hyperstimulation syndrome, symptoms from which can be categorized as mild, moderate, or severe
- Rupture or torsion of an ovarian cyst
- Ovarian malignancy

A2.

Ovarian hyperstimulation syndrome complicates pharmacological ovarian stimulation (ovarian induction therapy) as part of assisted reproduction techniques for the treatment of infertility. Rarely, it may arise spontaneously in pregnancy. Massive ovarian enlargement is due to multiple hormone-secreting luteinized ovarian cysts. Vascular dysfunction is manifested by arteriolar vasodilatation and increased capillary permeability, resulting in accumulation of fluid in pericardial and pleural cavities, leading to haemoconcentration and hypovolaemia. Ascites can lead to an abdominal compartment syndrome, with reduced cardiac output, reduced urine output, increased systemic vascular resistance, and coagulopathy.

A3.

Management may include:

- Bed rest
- Fluid replacement, either oral (guided by thirst) or intravenous. Intravenous colloids may be indicated with haemoconcentration and removal of large volumes of ascitic fluid
- Ascitic tap
- Thromboembolism prophylaxis
- Termination of pregnancy is very rarely needed

The syndrome is usually self-limiting and management is symptomatic and supportive, often on an outpatient basis.

Further Reading

RCOG. *The Management of Ovarian Hyperstimulation Syndrome.* Green-top Guideline No.5. 2016. Available from: https://www.rcog.org.uk/en/guidelines-research-services/guidelines/gtg5/

SAQ 5 **Pre-eclampsia-2**

A 38-year-old lady presents with headache. She is 36 weeks pregnant. You are concerned she may have pre-eclampsia.

Q1. List three signs or symptoms you would look out for to confirm your diagnosis.

Q2. The patient has a generalized seizure. What is your definitive treatment?

Q3. List three features of severe pre-eclampsia.

Answers

A1.

Pre-eclampsia is recognized by the presence of:

- New onset of hypertension—systolic blood pressure ≥140 mm Hg; diastolic blood pressure ≥90 mm Hg
- Proteinuria ≥300 mg in 24 hours; or urine dipstick protein 1+ or greater
- Generalized oedema, with swelling of the face, hands, and feet

It typically occurs after 20 weeks of pregnancy.

A2.

The treatment of choice is intravenous magnesium sulfate 4 g as a loading dose over 5 minutes, followed by an infusion of 1 G/hour maintained for 24 hours. Magnesium is an NMDA (N-methyl D-aspartate) receptor blocker, reversing cerebral vasoconstriction

A3.

Severe pre-eclampsia can be recognized by:

- Severe hypertension: systolic blood pressure ≥160 mm Hg; diastolic blood pressure ≥110 mm Hg
- Severe headache
- New onset visual disturbance, such as blurring of vision or flashing lights
- Right upper quadrant or epigastric abdominal pain due to liver distension, which is associated with liver tenderness and elevation in liver transaminases to at least twice the upper limit of normal
- Pulmonary oedema
- Papilloedema
- Signs of clonus
- Thrombocytopenia (platelet count less than 100 000/µL)
- HELLP syndrome (**H**aemolysis, **E**levated **L**iver enzymes, and **L**ow **P**latelet count)

Further Reading

Leslie D, Collis RE. Hypertension in pregnancy. *BJA Education*. 2016;16:33–7.

NICE. *Hypertension in Pregnancy: Diagnosis and Management CG107*. 2011. Available from: https://www.nice.org.uk/guidance/cg107

SAQ 6 **Endometrial Carcinoma**

A 47-year-old lady presents with heavy vaginal bleeding. She is worried she might have endometrial cancer, as she knows someone who died of this condition.

Q1. List four causes of abnormal uterine bleeding.
Q2. Give two risk factors for endometrial cancer.
Q3. How would you confirm the diagnosis?

Answers

A1.

Possible causes of abnormal uterine bleeding include:

- Structural abnormalities of the uterus: endometrial polyps; endometrial hyperplasia; fibroids; adenomyosis
- Cervical and endometrial malignancies
- Infections: cervicitis; endometritis
- Endocrine causes: hypothyroidism and hyperthyroidism; oestrogen producing tumours
- Haematological causes: coagulopathy
- Dysfunctional uterine bleeding: in the absence of pelvic pathology, pregnancy, or general medical disease

A2.

Multiple risk factors for endometrial carcinoma are recognized. A mnemonic is COLD NUT:

- **C**ancer (previous ovarian or breast cancers raise risk)
- **O**besity
- **L**ate menopause
- **D**iabetes
- **N**ulliparity
- **U**nopposed oestrogen (hormone replacement therapy, polycystic ovarian syndrome, anovulation)
- **T**amoxifen

A3.

A combined approach utilizing transvaginal ultrasound (to assess for heterogeneity and endometrial wall thickness) with endometrial biopsy is used to confirm the diagnosis.

Further Reading

Albers JR, Hull SK, Wesley RM. Abnormal uterine bleeding. *American Family Physician*. 2004;69:1915–26.

SAQ 7 **Ectopic Pregnancy**

A 34-year-old lady attends with intermittent vaginal bleeding for the last 24 hours. Her last menstrual period was 8 weeks ago. She has mild abdominal pain. She did a home pregnancy test, which was positive. A urine sample in the emergency department confirms the pregnancy. Her haemoglobin is 12.3 G/dl.

Q1. List four risk factors for ectopic pregnancy.

Q2. While you are assessing her, she becomes bradycardic and hypotensive and collapses. What is the likely mechanism and what should you do next?

Q3. Ultrasound shows an ectopic pregnancy. Her partner wants to know what are the chances of this recurring and what are the chances of her getting pregnant again?

Answers

A1.

Risk factors for ectopic pregnancy include:

- Previous ectopic pregnancy
- Previous PID
- Previous tubal surgery or ligation
- Assisted reproduction
- Increasing age (>35 years)
- Progesterone-only oral contraceptive pill
- Conception with intrauterine contraceptive device *in situ*

A2.

The likely mechanism for cardiovascular collapse is vagal stimulation secondary to products of conception at the cervical os. Patient requires speculum examination and removal of any products or clots.

A3.

There is a 25–30% chance of a further ectopic pregnancy, alongside a 60% chance of natural conception.

Further Reading

Diagnosis and management of ectopic pregnancy: green-top guideline no. 21. *BJOG*. 2016;123:e15–e55.

SAQ 8 **Ectopic Pregnancy 2**

A 26-year-old woman, who thinks she might be pregnant, presents with abdominal pain and vaginal bleeding and is noted to have tachycardia on examination. You are concerned that this might be an ectopic pregnancy.

Q1. How would you confirm the diagnosis?
Q2. Her serum βHCG is 998 U/L. Would you expect an intrauterine pregnancy be visualized on transvaginal ultrasound?
Q3. What are the options for treatment of an ectopic pregnancy?

Answers

A1.

Ectopic pregnancy is diagnosed using ultrasound, either transabdominal or transvaginal—the latter being the approach of choice. The features indicating ectopic pregnancy include:

- An empty uterine cavity, although an echogenic decidual cast or a pseudo-gestational sac (intrauterine fluid) may be seen
- Complex adnexal cyst or mass, which may contain a yolk sac or a living embryo
- Tubal ring sign or bagel sign of an echogenic ring surrounding an unruptured tubal pregnancy
- Ring of fire sign on colour Doppler, caused by hypervascularity around an adnexal mass
- Free fluid in the Pouch of Douglas

The finding of an intrauterine gestation sac almost always excludes ectopic pregnancy.

A2.

No. Generally a level of between 1500 and 2000 U/L is required before a sonographer can visualize an intrauterine pregnancy. A rise of just over 50% in 2 days suggests the pregnancy is viable and intra-uterine. Care must be taken however as some ectopic pregnancies can follow the β-HCG curve of a normal pregnancy. β HCG levels rise in a curvilinear fashion in early pregnancy, reaching a plateau at 9–11 weeks.

A3.

The treatment options for ectopic pregnancy include:

- Expectant management
- Methotrexate therapy
- Surgical management, which may be emergency surgery for a ruptured ectopic pregnancy, or planned laparoscopic surgery, and involves salpingectomy

Further Reading

Barash J, Buchanan EM, Hillson C. Diagnosis and management of ectopic pregnancy. *American Family Physician.* 2014;90:34–40.

SAQ 9 **Antepartum Haemorrhage**

A 32-year-old female who is 25 weeks pregnant attends the emergency department with abdominal and back pain, contractions, and vaginal bleeding. Her uterus is tender on examination. She has a blood pressure of 100/50 mm Hg, pulse rate 130 bpm, respiratory rate 23, and oxygen saturation of 99% on room air. She is on oxygen, and the paramedics have placed an intravenous cannula. Fluids are running.

Q1. Give four causes of antepartum haemorrhage, indicating which is most likely in this case.
Q2. What two investigations (which can be done at the bedside) would be most useful in determining the best course of management of this lady?
Q3. List four risk factors for this condition.

Answers

A1.

Causes of antepartum haemorrhage include:

- Placental abruption (separation of a normally sited placenta). This is characterized by painful vaginal bleeding with dark and non-clotting blood, abdominal tenderness, a hard and 'woody' uterus, uterine irritability, and abnormal uterine contractions. Abdominal and back pain and hypovolaemic shock out of proportion to visible blood loss indicate concealed haemorrhage.
- Placenta praevia (implantation of the placenta in the lower uterine segment), which may be associated with increasing degrees of placental invasion into the myometrium exemplified by placenta accreta, placenta increta, and placenta percreta. This usually presents with painless vaginal bleeding.
- Vasa praevia (fetal vessels).
- Local causes in the cervix or vagina such as cervical polyps, ectropion, or carcinoma, and vaginal varices.
- Trauma.

A2.

Bedside investigations for antepartum haemorrhage include:

- Ultrasound—confirms location of placenta, and demonstrates fetal lie and presentation and volume of liquor; 50% of abruptions are seen. Digital vaginal or rectal examination is contraindicated until placenta praevia can be excluded
- Cardiotocographic monitoring of fetal heart rate to check for fetal distress

A3.

Risk factors for antepartum haemorrhage are:

- Trauma
- Cocaine use
- Polyhydramnios

- Hypertension
- Pre-eclampsia/eclampsia/HELLP
- Premature rupture of membranes
- Thrombophilia
- Previous placental abruption
- Increasing maternal age
- High parity
- Chorioamnionitis
- Smoking during pregnancy

Further Reading

RCOG. *Antepartum Haemorrhage*. Green-top Guideline No.63. 2011. Available from: https://www.rcog.org.uk/en/guidelines-research-services/guidelines/gtg63/

SAQ 10 **Antepartum Haemorrhage 2**

A 26-year-old female, who is 30 weeks pregnant, is brought into the emergency department unresponsive in cardiac arrest with pulseless electrical activity. She is bleeding per vaginam. You suspect a catastrophic antepartum haemorrhage.

Q1. How does the management of cardiac arrest differ in this case?
Q2. What haematological complication often accompanies this condition?
Q3. What medication can be given to the mother to improve fetal outcome if delivered at this gestation (aside from standard resuscitation)?

Answers

A1.

The main differences are:

- Place patient in the left lateral position to move the uterus away from the inferior vena cava, preventing aorto-caval compression. This can be achieved by a 15–30 degree left lateral tilt (i.e. right side up), placement of a wedge under the right buttock and hip, or manual lateral displacement of the uterus to the left
- Need to proceed to emergency delivery within 5 minutes

A2.

Disseminated intravascular coagulation may often complicate antepartum haemorrhage. More than 50% of abruptions develop some degree of consumptive coagulopathy.

A3.

Steroids improve lung maturity and reduce incidence of necrotizing enterocolitis and intraventricular haemorrhage.

Further Reading

Walfish M, Neuman A, Wlody D. Maternal haemorrhage. *BJA*. 2009;103:Supplement 1: i47–i56.

SAQ 11 **Pelvic Pain**

A 35-year-old female attends with acute right-sided pelvic pain. She has had some milky vaginal discharge, but no dysuria. She is sexually active, and has normal menstrual periods. She is febrile (39°C), with a pulse rate of 110 beats per minute, and blood pressure 100/50 mm Hg. On abdominal examination there is tenderness in the right lower quadrant, with marked cervical excitation and right adnexal tenderness.

Q1. Give six possible causes of acute pelvic pain in this patient.
Q2. You make a diagnosis of PID. What are the two commonest causative organisms?
Q3. What treatment regime is indicated?

Answers

A1.

Causes of acute pelvic pain include:

- PID
- Ectopic pregnancy
- Ruptured ovarian cyst/twisted ovarian cyst
- Pyelonephritis
- Appendicitis
- Diverticulitis

A2.

The two commonest causative organisms are:

- Chlamydia
- *Neisseria gonorrhoeae*

A3.

Antibiotic treatment may involve:

- If being admitted: ceftriaxone 2 g intravenous, metronidazole 500 mg intravenous and doxycycline 100 mg oral; plus intravenous fluids
- If being discharged: ceftriaxone 500 mg intramuscular (or intravenous) then oral metronidazole and doxycycline

Further Reading

British Association for Sexual Health and HIV. *UK National Guideline for the Management of Pelvic Inflammatory Disease 2011 Clinical Effectiveness Group*. 2011. Available from: https://www.bashh.org/guidelines

SAQ 12 **Early Pregnancy Bleeding**

A 23-year-old female, G2 P1, presents to the emergency department with vaginal bleeding and passage of clots. She is 14 weeks pregnant. Her vital signs are: pulse rate 110 beats per minute, blood pressure 90/60 mm of mercury, respiratory rate 24 per minute, and SpO_2 98% on room air.

Q1. List three causes of haemodynamic stability associated with early pregnancy bleeding.
Q2. What clinical examinations should be performed? List two.
Q3. List three therapeutic interventions that can be considered or commenced while in the emergency department.

Answers

A1.

Haemodynamic instability can be associated with one of the following:

- Ruptured ectopic pregnancy
- Massive haemorrhage secondary to miscarriage
- Incomplete miscarriage with cervical shock, mediated by vagal stimulation secondary to products of conception in the cervical os
- Miscarriage with infection, leading to septic shock

A2.

Clinical assessment includes:

- Speculum examination, which allows recognition of cervical dilatation, and of local non-obstetric causes of bleeding, such as polyps, cervicitis, or carcinoma of the cervix
- Digital vaginal examination allows for palpation of the cervical os

A3.

Therapeutic interventions that can be commenced in the emergency department include:

- Venous access, with blood sent for grouping and cross matching, and crystalloid fluid infusion.
- Removal of products of conception at the cervical os via a speculum; the material should be sent for histopathological examination.
- Anti-D immunoglobulin for all Rhesus-negative non-sensitized women. Anti-D is currently recommended for all spontaneous miscarriage, complete or incomplete, at or after 12 weeks' gestation, and where surgical evacuation of the uterus is carried out. 250 IU is administered within 72 hours, or 500 IU after 20 weeks.

Further Reading

NICE. *Ectopic Pregnancy and Miscarriage. Diagnosis and Initial Management in Early Pregnancy of Ectopic Pregnancy and Miscarriage, CG154.* 2012. Available from:
RCOG. *The Use of Anti-D Immunoglobulin for Rhesus D Prophylaxis.* Green-top Guideline No 22. 2011. Available from: https://www.rcog.org.uk/en/guidelines-research-services/guidelines/gtg22/

SAQ 13 **Abdominal Trauma in Pregnancy**

A 27-year-old female, G3 P2, who is 20 weeks' pregnant, attends the emergency department following a road traffic collision. She was driving a car, which went into the back of another car at 40 miles per hour. She was wearing a seat belt, and the air bags did not deploy. She complains of abdominal pain. Her vital signs are pulse rate 100 beats per minute, blood pressure 124/70 mm of mercury, respiratory rate 20 per minute, and SpO_2 on room air 100%.

Q1. List three obstetric complications of blunt abdominal trauma in pregnancy.
Q2. What assessments would you consider in the emergency department? List two.
Q3. List three clinical features of uterine rupture.

Answers

A1.

Obstetric complications of abdominal trauma include:

- Placental abruption
- Feto-maternal transfusion, which may lead to sensitization in Rhesus-negative women
- Preterm labour
- Premature rupture of membranes
- Uterine rupture
- Amniotic fluid embolism

A2.

Assessments to be considered in the emergency department include:

- Ultrasound evaluation of the fetus
- Fetal heart rate monitoring
- Blood typing to identify Rhesus type
- Imaging of the abdomen, which may include ultrasound and/or computed tomography (CT) scanning. The fetal radiation dose for CT examinations usually does not exceed a threshold of 50 mGy (5 rad). Radiological advice can be sought for the calculation of estimated fetal radiation dose. In general, radiological studies that are indicated for maternal evaluation should not be delayed due to concerns about fetal radiation exposure

A3.

Uterine rupture is characterized by:

- Severe abdominal pain
- Guarding and rebound tenderness
- Abnormal fetal lie, which may be oblique or transverse

- Easily palpated fetal parts
- Smaller than expected fundal height for period of gestation
- Absent fetal heart sounds

Further Reading

Jain V, Chari R, Maslovitz S, Farine D, Maternal Fetal Medicine Committee, Bujold E, et al. Guidelines for the management of a pregnant trauma patient *Journal of Obstetrics and Gynaecology Canada*. 2015;37:553–71.
Murphy NJ, Quinlan JD. Trauma in pregnancy: assessment, management and prevention *American Family Physician*. 2014;90:717–24.

Chapter 17 **Ophthalmology**

SAQ 1 **Acute Angle Closure Glaucoma**

A 72-year-old lady presents at 11.00 pm with left-sided headache and vomiting. There is no history of trauma. Her neurological examination is normal except for left-sided blurred vision. You note a red left eye with a dilated pupil.

Q1. What is the likely diagnosis?
Q2. What other signs or symptoms would you be looking for?
Q3. What treatment is indicated?

Answers

A1.

Acute angle closure glaucoma is the most likely diagnosis. It classically presents in the late evening or at night, when the pupil physiologically dilates in response to dim light. Susceptible individuals are those with shallow anterior chambers (the space between the iris and the cornea), which is often associated with cataract. Dilation of the pupil in dim lighting conditions causes the iris to bunch up at the periphery, occluding the drainage angle. With no drainage available, the pressure in the anterior chamber starts to rise. Under increasing pressure, the pupil is pushed posteriorly against the lens, causing pupil block. Pupil block prevents the normal flow of aqueous from behind the iris, through the pupil to its drainage site in the anterior chamber. Subsequently, aqueous being produced behind the iris is trapped, pushing the iris forwards, further narrowing the anterior chamber space, and closing the angle further. Once established in this cycle, pupil block can only be relieved by either constricting the pupil to draw the iris away from the peripheral angle or, more definitively, by creating a hole in the iris to allow direct passage of the aqueous from the posterior to the anterior chamber (peripheral iridotomy).

A2.

Acute angle closure glaucoma can present with an acutely painful, photophobic red eye, a cloudy cornea, fixed semi-dilated oval pupil, circumcorneal or ciliary redness, reduced pupillary reflex, a shallow anterior chamber (the iris bowing forwards), and a stony hard globe. The patient might describe blurred vision or profound reduction in visual acuity, and halos around bright lights. This is usually unilateral, but the unaffected eye is at risk of future attacks of acute glaucoma.

A3.

The best way to relieve the pain is to reduce the intraocular pressure. Reduce the production of aqueous by administering 500 mg acetazolamide (carbonic anhydrase inhibitor) intravenous as a bolus. One drop of 0.5% timolol (topical non-selective beta-blocker) further reduces the production of aqueous. Administration of 2% pilocarpine drops (cholinergic) may be used to constrict the pupil to facilitate drainage. The definite treatment by the ophthalmologist should be a bilateral laser peripheral iridotomy. This procedure provides an alternative pathway for drainage of the aqueous from the posterior chamber into the anterior chamber.

Further Reading

Khondkaryan A, Francis BA. *Angle-closure Glaucoma*. American Academy of Ophthalmology. 2013. Available from: https://www.aao.org/munnerlyn-laser-surgery-center/angleclosure-glaucoma-19

SAQ 2 **Orbital Cellulitis**

A six-year-old child attends the emergency department with his mother. The mother is concerned as she noted his left eyelid to be swollen, red, and painful. The child has been otherwise well.

Q1. You think this child might have preseptal cellulitis. What are the red flag signs for orbital cellulitis?
Q2. What is the most common bacteria causative of orbital cellulitis?
Q3. What investigation would you perform if concerned about orbital cellulitis?

Answers

A1.

Signs that could suggest orbital cellulitis would be rapid onset and progression, high fever, severe ocular pain, reduced visual acuity, intense eyelid swelling, congested conjunctival and episcleral vessels, chemosis (conjunctival oedema), proptosis, painful or restricted eye movements (ophthalmoplegia), afferent pupillary defect, forehead anaesthesia, and optic nerve dysfunction. NB: young children (under age of five) are more at risk of developing orbital cellulitis from preseptal (periorbital) cellulitis and therefore must be treated aggressively (either intravenous antibiotics or oral antibiotics with daily review).

A2.

The most common causative bacterial organisms in orbital cellulitis are:

- *Staphylococcus aureus*
- *Streptococcus pneumoniae*
- *Streptococcus pyogenes* (beta-haemolytic streptococcus)
- Others include *Enterococcus*, *Klebsiella*, and *Haemophilus influenzae* type B

A3.

A computed tomography (CT) scan of the orbit and sinuses with contrast is the most important investigation: paranasal sinus disease is the most common infective origin of orbital cellulitis and therefore needs to be identified, as surgical drainage by the ear, nose, throat (ENT) surgeon is necessary for treatment. CT scans may show inflammatory stranding in the intraconal fat, intraconal soft tissue mass, oedema of extraocular muscles, and subperiosteal abscess formation, along with evidence of paranasal sinus disease.

Further Reading

Lee S, Yen MT. Management of preseptal and orbital cellulitis. *Saudi Journal of Ophthalmology*. 2011;25:21–9.

SAQ 3 **Orbital Cellulitis 2**

A 13-year-old presents with swelling and redness to the eyelid and cheek. Your junior colleague has seen the patient and is worried that this might be orbital cellulitis.

Q1. What is the anatomical difference between preseptal cellulitis and orbital cellulitis?

Q2. How can you differentiate clinically between preseptal cellulitis and orbital cellulitis?

Q3. You decide this is preseptal cellulitis. What follow-up plan would you implement?

Answers

A1.

Preseptal (periorbital) cellulitis is a condition where there is infection and inflammation of the eyelid which is superficial and confined to the soft tissues which are superficial to the orbital septum. The orbital septum is a fibrous membrane which separates the orbital fat from the eyelid fat and levator palpebrae superioris. Orbital cellulitis involves the orbital soft tissues which are involved in ocular function and usually is caused by bacterial sinusitis. It, unlike preseptal cellulitis, warrants urgent imaging and evaluation by both an ophthalmologist and a head-and-neck consultant because it has much more associated morbidity.

A2.

Features more suggestive of orbital cellulitis are:

• High fever
• Ocular pain
• Pain on eye movement
• Proptosis
• Chemosis
• Visual disturbance

A3.

Preseptal cellulitis in children can be managed on an outpatient basis on oral antibiotics; however daily follow-up is required. Adults can be seen less frequently unless there is any concern over progression in which case it must also be daily. Those admitted with suspected orbital cellulitis need to be started on intravenous broad-spectrum antibiotics and monitored closely. As they improve, they can eventually be stepped down to oral antibiotics.

Further Reading

Sadovsky R. Distinguishing periorbital from orbital cellulitis. *American Family Physician*. 2003;67:1349–53.

SAQ 4 **Horner's Syndrome**

A 72-year-old male presents to your department complaining of a cough and lethargy. On examination, you notice the following features as shown in Fig. 17.1.

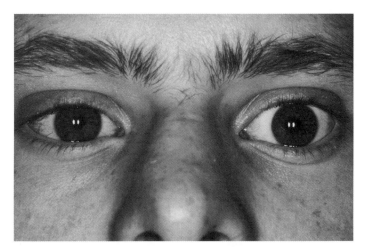

Fig. 17.1 Reproduced with permission from Wilkinson, I. et al. (2017). *Oxford Handbook of Clinical Medicine.* 10th ed. Oxford University Press. © Oxford University Press 2017. Reproduced with permission of the licensor via PLSClear.

Q1. What is the diagnosis?
Q2. What are the clinical features of this diagnosis?
Q3. List three anatomical sites which may be affected thereby giving rise to the diagnosis?

Answers

A1.

The diagnosis is Horner's syndrome, due to a lesion of the ipsilateral oculosympathetic pathway first described in 1869 by the Swiss ophthalmologist Johann Friedrich Horner.

A2.

Clinical features of Horner's syndrome are:

- Miosis, leading to anisocoria (difference in pupillary size)
- Anhidrosis (loss of sweating in one half of the face)
- Partial ptosis of the upper eyelid, less than 2 mm (due to paralysis of Muller's muscle in the upper eyelid)
- Enophthalmos

Horner's syndrome is an excellent lateralizing, but a poor localizing, sign.

A3.

Lesions causing Horner's syndrome may be located in:

- Lower brain stem (associated with bulbar signs), associated with the reticular formation (e.g. lateral medullary syndrome)
- Lower cervical and upper thoracic spinal cord at C8-T1 levels (associated with myelopathic signs), associated with sympathetic preganglionic neurons (e.g. trauma, myelitis, neoplasm, infarction, syringomyelia)
- First thoracic nerve root (e.g. brachial plexus trauma)
- Apex of the lung (e.g. Pancoast syndrome)
- Internal carotid artery (e.g. dissection, aneurysm)
- Cavernous sinus (e.g. thrombosis, mass; carotid-cavernous fistula)
- Apex of the orbit

SAQ 5 **Orbital Fractures**

During the early hours of Saturday morning a 19-year-old male presents with a friend, slightly intoxicated, and with significant bruising and swelling to his face around the left eye. He tells you he 'walked into a wall', to which his similarly intoxicated friend laughs.

Q1. What is the most common pattern of injury with an orbital fracture?
Q2. What are the two main concerning complications of an orbital fracture?
Q3. Which patient group is most at risk?

Answers

A1.

Most commonly the fracture involves the zygomatico-maxillary complex, which includes the zygoma and lateral orbital wall (associated with malar or cheekbone impact). The next most common types are the naso-orbito-ethmoidal fractures (associated with central upper mid-face impact) followed by internal orbital or orbital wall fractures (blow in and blow out fractures), such as orbital floor, medial wall, or roof fractures. In around half of cases, where the orbital wall is involved, more than one wall is fractured.

A2.

Due to the very thin nature of the orbital floor, a fracture here (known as a pure 'blow out' fracture when caused by blunt trauma to the globe) can cause a hole allowing the soft tissues of the orbit to herniate through. The level of the globe can drop (hypoglobus) and sink back into the socket (enophthalmos). The two concerns in this fracture pattern are:

- Risk of Volkmann's ischaemic contracture of the inferior rectus which may have become trapped (failure of upward gaze, associated with pain and diplopia)
- Oculovagal syndrome due to the entrapped inferior rectus. Oculovagal syndrome occurs due to the tension on the inferior rectus muscle. The mechanism of this is via afferent trigeminal ophthalmic sensory fibres which communicate via the ascending reticular formation with vagal efferent fibres. Symptoms and signs may include bradycardia, hypotension, headaches, nausea/vomiting, and it may even be life-threatening. Sometimes only nausea and vomiting are experienced which can be mistakenly attributed to head injury.

A3.

Children are most at risk of these complications as their relatively elastic skeleton makes a 'trap-door' fracture complex more likely, thus trapping the inferior rectus muscle. If this is not released in 24–48 hours, then irreversible ischaemia, contracture, and then irreversible mobility derangement is possible.

Further Reading

Joseph JM, Glavas IP. Orbital fractures: a review. *Clinical Ophthalmology*. 2011;5:95–100.

SAQ 6 **Retinal Vein Occlusion**

An 87-year-old woman presents with a two-day history of increasing difficulty to read. Her visual acuity is considerably reduced. You see the following view on fundoscopy in Fig. 17.2.

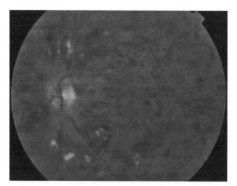

Fig. 17.2 Reproduced with permission from Sundaram, V. et al. (2016). *Training in Ophthalmology*. 2nd ed. Oxford University Press. © Oxford University Press 2016. Reproduced with permission of the licensor via PLSClear.

Q1. What is the diagnosis on fundoscopy?
Q2. Describe three findings on this image.
Q3. Give three risk factors for the causative condition.

Answers

A1.

Central retinal vein occlusion (CRVO), which is the second most common retinal vascular disease after diabetic retinopathy and typically occurs in patients aged 50 years or over, with an equal sex distribution. It presents with sudden painless unilateral loss of vision or distortion of vision.

A2.

Any of the following are indicative of CRVO: 'stormy sunset appearance', engorged and tortuous retinal veins, flame shaped haemorrhages (which involve all four quadrants of the retina), cotton wool spots, and disc oedema. Fluorescein angiography will demonstrate capillary non-perfusion in all four quadrants of the retina.

A3.

Any of the following: older age, hypertension, hyperlipidaemia, diabetes mellitus, thrombophilia, glaucoma, and coagulopathies are risk factors.

Further Reading

NICE. *Ranibizumab for the Treatment of Macular Oedema Caused by Retinal Vein Occlusion (RVO)*. 2011. Available from: https://www.nice.org.uk/guidance/ta283/documents/macular-oedema-retinal-vein-occlusion-ranibizumab-erg-report2

Royal College of Ophthalmologists. *Clinical Guidelines: Retinal Vein Occlusion (RVO)*. 2015. Available from: https://www.rcophth.ac.uk/wp-content/uploads/2015/07/Retinal-Vein-Occlusion-RVO-Guidelines-July-2015.pdf

SAQ 7 **Central Retinal Artery Occlusion**

A 72-year-old man presents to the emergency department with a sudden painless loss of vision in his left eye. You see the following view on fundoscopy in Fig. 17.3.

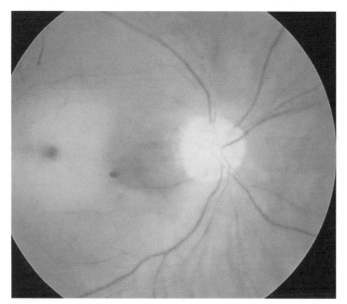

Fig. 17.3 Reproduced with permission from Sundaram, V. et al. (2016). *Training in Ophthalmology*. 2nd ed. Oxford University Press. © Oxford University Press 2016. Reproduced with permission of the licensor via PLSClear.

Q1. What is the diagnosis?

Q2. Give three risk factors for developing this condition.

Q3. What is the suggested initial treatment while awaiting review by the ophthalmologist?

Answers

A1.

Central retinal artery occlusion, which is analogous to an acute ocular stroke. Note the classic appearance of cherry spot macula: the pale retina (supplied by retinal arterial) and the perfused macula (supplied by the choroid/posterior ciliary arteries).

A2.

Any of the following are risk factors: hypertension; atrial fibrillation; hyperlipidaemia; smoking; diabetes mellitus; coagulopathy; plus any other risk factors for an embolus (e.g. cardiac valvular disease).

A3.

Digital massage of the globe through the closed eyelids for 10–15 seconds at a time, over a period of 10–15 minutes. The massage is believed to potentially dislodge the thrombus. Other temporization treatment options (all aim to reduce intraocular pressure) include intravenous acetazolamide 500 mg (carbonic anhydrase inhibitor) or sublingual glyceryl trinitrate puffs.

Further Reading

Olsen TW, Pulido JS, Folk JC, Hyman L, Flaxel CJ, Adelman RA. *Retinal and Ophthalmic Artery Occlusions Preferred Practice Pattern.* Available from: http://dx.doi.org/10.1016/j.ophtha.2016.09.024

SAQ 8 **Vitreous Haemorrhage**

A 45-year-old diabetic male attends the emergency department with painless visual loss in his left eye. A few days ago, he noted occasional floaters. His visual acuity is down to 6/12 in his left eye. You see the following view on fundoscopy in Fig. 17.4.

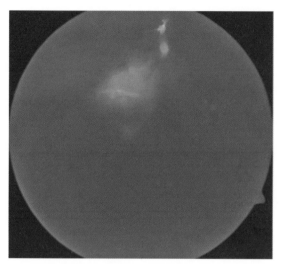

Fig. 17.4 Reproduced with permission from Sundaram, V. et al. (2016). *Training in Ophthalmology*. 2nd ed. Oxford University Press. © Oxford University Press 2016. Reproduced with permission of the licensor via PLSClear.

Q1. What is the diagnosis?
Q2. Other than diabetes mellitus, give two more risk factors.
Q3. List three complications.

Answers

A1.

Vitreous haemorrhage, which is the extravasation of blood into and around the vitreous humor (vitreous chamber).

A2.

Risk factors for vitreous haemorrhage include old age (age-related macular degeneration), posterior vitreous detachment, retinal detachment or tear, central or branch retinal vein occlusion, hypertension, sickle cell retinopathy, ocular trauma, and non-accidental injury (shaken baby syndrome). Proliferative diabetic retinopathy is the main risk factor due to weak vessels formed during neovascularization.

A3.

Vitreous haemorrhage may be complicated by glaucoma; proliferative vitreoretinopathy; haemosiderosis bulbi.

Further Reading

American Academy of Ophthalmology. *Vitreous Hemorrhage: Diagnosis and Treatment*. 2007. Available from: https://www.aao.org/eyenet/article/vitreous-hemorrhage-diagnosis-treatment-2

SAQ 9 **Intraocular Foreign Body**

A 45-year-old metal worker has presented to the emergency department with pain, lacrimation, photophobia, and foreign body sensation in the left eye. Symptoms initially developed when he was using an angle grinder, three hours previously. He was not wearing his usual eye protection. You suspect a foreign body in the eye.

Q1. List three assessments you would consider in the emergency department.
Q2. How would you treat a corneal foreign body?
Q3. List three recommendations for care following treatment.

Answers

A1.

Three initial assessments include:

- Documentation of visual acuity
- Fluorescein staining of the cornea and observation with a blue light
- Slit lamp examination to localize and characterize the foreign body
- Imaging for suspected intraocular injuries: anteroposterior and lateral x-rays of the orbit in up and down gaze; CT scan

A2.

A corneal foreign body can be removed under topical anaesthesia (e.g. tetracaine) using a sterile green (21 gauge) hypodermic needle under slit lamp magnification, with the patient focusing on a distant object and the operator's hand resting on the patient's cheek for stabilization. The foreign body is approached tangentially and dislodged using a flicking motion. Irrigation of the eye or use of a moistened cotton-tipped applicator are generally not useful.

A3.

- Provision of antibiotic eye drops or ointment
- A topical cycloplegic may relieve pain by reducing ciliary spasm
- Follow-up to ensure healing and resolution of associated rust ring
- Eye patching is not beneficial
- Provide advice on wearing of eye protection to prevent a recurrent injury

Further Reading

Ahmed E, House RJ. Feldman corneal abrasions and corneal foreign bodies. *Primary Health Care*. 2015;42:363–75.
Aslam SA, Sheth HG, Vaughan AJ. Emergency management of corneal injuries. *Injury*. 2007;38:594–7.

SAQ 10 **Perforating Injury of the Eye**

You have been asked to see a 22-year-old male who is the victim of assault. He has extensive swelling around the right eye and a deep laceration of the upper eyelid. You are concerned about the possibility of a perforating injury of the globe of the eye.

Q1. There is extensive eyelid swelling. How can you improve visualization of the eye?
Q2. List four signs of perforating injury of the globe of the eye.
Q3. List three treatments you would initiate in the emergency department.

Answers

A1.

Visualization of the eye can be improved by the use of lid retractors in the presence of massive eyelid swelling or blepharospasm. Inability to visualize the globe in the emergency department should warrant urgent ophthalmological consultation.

A2.

Signs of perforation of the globe include:

- Subconjunctival haemorrhage
- Conjunctival laceration
- Haemorrhagic chemosis
- Hyphaema (blood in the anterior chamber)
- Collapse of, or asymmetrical depth of, the anterior chamber
- An irregular pupil, which may be teardrop-shaped due to prolapse of the iris into the wound, or from iridodialysis (tear of the iris from the ciliary body)
- Seidel sign: appearance of a 'dark waterfall' clearing away fluorescein on the corneal surface caused by aqueous emission
- Reduced intraocular pressure, leading to a soft and hypotonic globe (this sign should not be sought actively)

A3.

The management of a perforating globe injury includes the following:

- A rigid eye shield should be taped in place
- Any protruding foreign body should be stabilized
- Intravenous antibiotic therapy

- Antiemetic
- Review of tetanus prophylaxis
- Urgent referral to an ophthalmologist

Further Reading

Harlan JB, Jr, Pieramici DJ. Evaluation of patients with ocular trauma. *Ophthalmology Clinics of North America.* 2002;15:153–61.

SAQ 11 **Chemical Injury to the Cornea**

A 37-year-old man has been working on a ceiling and felt some fragments of plaster go into his eyes. He has had a washout of both eyes at the scene, but has continued symptoms. Your assessment is that he has sustained an alkaline injury to the eyes.

Q1. What immediate measures need to be carried out in the emergency department?
Q2. List clinical features suggestive of alkaline injury to the cornea.
Q3. List three complications of alkaline injury to the eye.

Answers

A1.

Immediate irrigation of conjunctival sac should be commenced with sterile water or normal saline, aided by topical anaesthesia and a lid speculum, until pH is neutral (7.4), as measured using universal indicator paper, or equal to that in the unexposed eye. This may be aided by an intravenous delivery system and a Morgan contact lens. Irrigate the whole eye, including under the upper and lower eyelids. Deliver a minimum of 2 litres or until normal pH is restored.

Particulate material should be removed from the conjunctival fornices with a cotton-tipped applicator, aided by double eversion of the upper eyelid for removal from the upper fornix.

The cornea should be stained with fluorescein to allow assessment for epithelial defects using the slit lamp.

A2.

Signs suggestive of corneal injury include:

- Conjunctival injection or blanching, chemosis, haemorrhage, epithelial defects
- Corneal epitheliopathy: punctuate to complete loss of epithelium, corneal oedema
- Perilimbal ischaemia with blanching of vessels
- Anterior chamber reaction

A3.

Complications of ocular alkaline injury include:

- Corneal ulceration; recurrent corneal abrasions
- Corneal scarring leading to opacification and neovascularization
- Symblepharon (adhesions between the eyelids and the globe)
- Secondary glaucoma and cataract

Further Reading

Hemmati HD, Colby KA. Treating acute chemical injuries of the cornea. *EyeNet*. 2012;9: 42–5.

SAQ 12 **Orbital Compartment Syndrome**

A 50-year-old male presents with severe pain in, and proptosis of, the right eye following blunt trauma. There is a strong likelihood of retrobulbar haemorrhage, leading to acute increase in orbital pressure.

Q1. What clinical features suggest retrobulbar haemorrhage? List four.
Q2. Prior to transfer to a specialist ophthalmological centre, what treatment can be offered in the emergency department?
Q3. List three other causes of orbital compartment syndrome.

Answers

A1.

Features suggesting retrobulbar haemorrhage include:

- Acute and rapidly progressing loss of vision
- Tense proptosis
- Diffuse subconjunctival haemorrhage with posterior extension
- Ophthalmoplegia
- Fixed dilated pupil with afferent pupillary defect
- Elevated intraocular pressure
- Fundoscopy may show retinal venous congestion and central retinal artery pulsations

A2.

Immediate decompression of the globe can be achieved by a lateral canthotomy and inferior cantholysis as a temporary measure under local anaesthesia (1% lidocaine with 1 in 200 000 adrenaline).

A3.

Orbital compartment syndrome may also be caused by:

- Orbital haemorrhage following surgery or retrobulbar injection, or related to coagulation disorder
- Orbital cellulitis
- Orbital emphysema
- Orbital tumours
- Orbital foreign bodies

Further Reading

Lima V, Burt B, Leibovitch I, Prabhakaran V, Goldberg RA, Selva D. Orbital compression syndrome: the ophthalmic surgical emergency. *Survey of Ophthalmology*. 2009;54:441–9.

Chapter 18 **Paediatrics**

SAQ 1 **Type I Diabetes Mellitus**

One of the CT1 doctors approaches you to discuss a child he is looking after in the paediatric area. He has a 5-year-old girl he is concerned about because he thinks she may have undiagnosed diabetes and may be presenting with diabetic ketoacidosis (DKA).

Q1. List six features in the history and/or examination which might alert you to the possibility of this diagnosis?
Q2. At what glucose level should DKA be suspected?
Q3. Outline the principles of fluid management in paediatric DKA.

Answers

A1.

The features of diabetic ketoacidosis include:

- polydipsia
- polyuria; nocturia; enuresis
- recent unexplained weight loss
- nausea/vomiting
- abdominal pain
- tiredness
- hyperventilation
- dehydration
- reduced level of consciousness

A2.

DKA should be suspected with a glucose level of 11 mmol/L or above.

Venous blood gas, urea and electrolytes, plus a capillary (or urinary) ketone measurement are also necessary to confirm the diagnosis. Diabetic ketoacidosis is possible with normal blood glucose levels. Euglycaemic DKA is associated with reduced carbohydrate intake leading to decreased gluconeogenesis.

A3.

Alert children, who are not clinically dehydrated, and not nauseous or vomiting, can be offered oral rehydration and subcutaneous insulin with regular monitoring of ketone levels, even though initial ketone levels are high.

No fluid (normal saline) bolus is indicated in mild or moderate diabetic ketoacidosis (DKA) with pH 7.1 or more.

Ideally no fluid bolus should be given in severe DKA (with pH less than 7.1), and no more than one bolus of 10 ml/kg 0.9% sodium chloride should be given without discussion with a senior paediatrician. If more than 20 ml/kg of fluid bolus is given, this amount should be subtracted from the calculated overall 48hour fluid volume requirement.

Total fluid for the first 48 hours is the estimated deficit plus the maintenance fluids:

- mild/moderate DKA with pH 7.1 or more = 5% deficit
- severe DKA with pH less than 7.1 = 10% deficit

Maintenance using 'reduced volume' rules to reduce the risk of cerebral oedema:

- weight <10 kg = 2 ml/kg/hour
- weight 10–40 kg = 1 ml/kg/hour
- weight >40 kg = 40 ml/hour

Deficit replacement over 48 hours is advised; 0.9% sodium chloride with 20 mmol KCl is the fluid of choice until the plasma glucose falls below 14 mmol/L. Overall local guidelines and protocols should be followed.

Further Reading

BSPED. *BSPED Recommended Guidelines for the Management of Children and Young People Under the Age of 18 Years with Diabetic Ketoacidosis.* 2015. Available from: https://www.bsped.org.uk/media/1381/dkaguideline.pdf

NICE. *Diabetes (Type 1 and Type 2) In Children and Young People: Diagnosis and Management NG18.* 2015. Available from: https://www.nice.org.uk/guidance/NG18

SAQ 2 **Diabetic Ketoacidosis**

A 12-year-old boy presents with abdominal pain, lethargy, and high blood sugar. You suspect diabetic ketoacidosis (DKA).

Q1. List two biochemical predictors of a poor outcome in diabetic ketoacidosis.
Q2. Give two ways in which the management differs from treatment of adult DKA.
Q3. What are the three main causes of mortality in children that present with diabetic ketoacidosis?

Answers

A1.

Poor outcome in DKA is predicted by:
   Venous pH <7.1, bicarbonate <5 mmol/L.

A2.

Differences between management of adult and paediatric DKA include the following:

* Intravenous insulin therapy is commenced at least one hour after commencement of intravenous fluid therapy
* Fluid boluses are not recommended
* Insulin by continuous low-dose infusion is only given when shock has been reversed
* Insulin boluses are contraindicated

The treatment is different because of the risk of cerebral oedema in children, and because the degree of dehydration is often overestimated. Large volumes of infused fluid are harmful. Cerebral oedema is the most common cause of death in paediatric ketoacidosis.

A3.

Causes of mortality in diabetic ketoacidosis include:

* Cerebral oedema, which is associated with headache, recurrent vomiting, drowsiness, restlessness and irritability, hypoxaemia, seizures, and neurological signs such as cranial nerve palsies, decorticate or decerebrate posturing, abnormal pupillary responses, and Cushing's triad (hypertension, bradycardia, and abnormal respiratory pattern)
* Aspiration pneumonia
* Hypokalaemia

Further Reading

BSPED. *BSPED Recommended Guidelines for the Management of Children and Young People Under the Age of 18 Years with Diabetic Ketoacidosis*. 2015. Available from: https://www.bsped.org.uk/media/1381/dkaguideline.pdf

SAQ 3 **Croup**

A two-year-old boy is brought to the emergency department at 10 pm with difficulty in breathing and a barking cough. The triage nurse suspects croup (laryngotracheobronchitis).

Q1. What is the first line treatment for croup in the emergency department?
Q2. Name a scoring system that aids in stratifying the severity of croup
Q3. What are the components of this score?

Answers

A1.

Initial therapy consists for croup consists of:

- Dexamethasone (accepted doses range from 0.15 mg/kg to 0.6 mg/kg) in a single dose, which is equally effective if administered by the oral, intravenous, or intramuscular routes. The oral route is preferred where oral intake is possible. Dexamethasone has a longer half-life and higher anti-inflammatory activity than prednisolone, providing therapeutic effects over the usual period of symptoms lasting 72 hours. Clinical improvement is seen within six hours of administration. It reduces the need for hospital admissions and for reattendance with continuing problems.
- Budesonide 2 mg nebulized is an alternative treatment option if oral dexamethasone can be tolerated due to vomiting.

The use of steroids reduces laryngeal oedema and the need for any additional medical therapy, such as nebulized adrenaline. Croup is usually a mild, benign, and self-limiting illness.

A2.

The Westley score enables stratification of severity of presentation with croup.

A3.

Components of the scoring system are:

- **C**yanosis
- **A**ir entry
- **R**etractions (intercostal recessions)
- **L**evel of consciousness
- **S**aturation <92%

Remember the acronym *CARLS* (it is unlikely you will be expected to know the exact scoring for each component).

Further Reading

Bjornson CL, Johnson DW. Croup in children. *CMAJ (Canadian Medical Association Journal)*. 2013;195:1317–23.

SAQ 4 **Intussusception**

A 15-month-old child presents to the emergency department following a three-day history of a viral illness with a maculopapular rash. On the day prior to presentation he had had bouts of colic but had been eating and drinking and had been otherwise settled. He looks unwell, with bloody diarrhoea and a capillary refill time of 3 seconds. His abdominal X-ray is shown in Fig. 18.1.

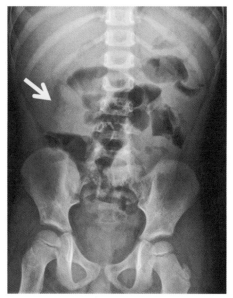

Fig. 18.1 Reproduced with permission from Reid, J. et al. (2013). *Pediatric Radiology*. Oxford University Press USA. © Oxford University Press 2013. Reproduced with permission of the licensor via PLSClear.

Q1. What is the likely diagnosis based on this abdominal X-ray?
Q2. List three predisposing factors.
Q3. Name two treatment options.

Answers

A1.

The diagnosis is intussusception. Plain abdominal X-rays may reveal an elongated soft tissue mass, coexisting with features of small bowel obstruction. There is absence of gas in the ascending colon, distal to the site of obstruction.

A2.

Predisposing factors for intussusception are:

- Recent viral illness
- Meckel's diverticulum
- Henoch–Schönlein purpura
- Intestinal polyps, as in Peutz–Jeghers syndrome
- Cystic fibrosis

A3.

Potential treatments include:

- Pneumatic insufflation with air enema
- Hydrostatic reduction with barium or water-soluble contrast enema
- Surgical reduction

Further Reading

Mandeville K, Chien M, Willyerd FA, Mandell G, Hostetler MA, Bulloch B. Intussusception: clinical presentations and imaging characteristics. *Pediatric Emergency Care*. 2012;28:842–4.

SAQ 5 **Resuscitation Scenario**

A prealert has been sent to the emergency department. A four-year-old boy has been knocked down by a car and is being brought to the emergency room.

Q1. As you anticipate arrival, show your calculation of his estimated body weight.
Q2. What tracheal tube diameter and length may be required for this patient?
Q3. What initial fluid bolus may be required?

Answers

A1.

Estimated body weight = (age in years + 4) × 2 kg = 16 kg.

A2.

Tracheal tube diameter = (age in years/4) + 4 mm = size 5.
   Tracheal tube length = (age/2) + 12 for oral intubation = 14 cm.

A3.

Calculated fluid bolus = 10 ml/kg crystalloid in trauma (10 ml/kg packed red cells in cases of extremis or where significant bleeding is suspected).

SAQ 6 **Croup 2**

The paediatric emergency department nurses ask you to come to see a child they think has croup.

Q1. What area of the airway is affected in croup?
Q2. What is the clinical feature which leads to the diagnosis of croup?
Q3. On examining the child, you notice the child has stridor on agitation, has some mild retractions, has normal air entry, oxygen saturations above 92% times and a normal level of consciousness. What would be their Westley score and how would this group them?

Answers

A1.

There is subglottic inflammation in acute viral laryngo-tracheobronchitis.

A2.

Croup is a clinical diagnosis. The clinical features of hoarse voice, 'barking' cough, and inspiratory stridor lead to consideration of the diagnosis of croup.

A3.

The Westley score is 2.
The Westley score is reproduced in Table 18.1.

Table 18.1

SCORE	Stridor	Retractions	Air entry	SaO$_2$ <92%	Level of consciousness
0	None	None	Normal	None	Normal
1	Upon agitation	Mild	Mild decrease		
2	At rest	Moderate	Marked decrease		
3		Severe			
4				Upon agitation	
5				At rest	Decreased

Mild (0–2) Moderate (3–5) Severe (6–11) Impending respiratory failure (12–17).
Oxygen should be given if saturations below 92% on room air. Nebulized adrenaline would only be indicated in the severe/life threatening cases. Oral dexamethasone is the preferred treatment in the first instance.
Reproduced with permission from Marsh, A. (2014). Croup - RCEMLearning. [online] RCEMLearning. Available at: https://www.rcemlearning.co.uk/references/croup/ [Accessed 22 Jan. 2019].

Further Reading

Westley CR, Cotton EK, Brooks JG. Nebulized racemic epinephrine by IPPB for the treatment of croup: a double-blind study *American Journal of Diseases of Childhood.* 1978;132(5):484–7.

SAQ 7 **Gastroenteritis**

A 20-month-old girl presents to the department with her parents, who are concerned as she has developed vomiting and diarrhoea this evening.

Q1. Give three risk factors, in children, for the development of dehydration.

Q2. In which three circumstances should stool samples be requested?

Q3. Following specialist advice, in which circumstances might antibiotics be considered?

Answers

A1.

Risk factors for the development of dehydration include:

- Age: less than one and more specifically less than six months of age
- Low birthweight infants
- Passage of greater than five diarrhoeal stools in the preceding 24 hours
- More than two episodes of vomiting in the preceding 24 hours
- Not having been offered (or able to tolerate) fluids prior to presenting
- Cessation of breastfeeding during the illness
- Signs of malnutrition

A2.

A stool sample should be requested for microbiological analysis:

- If there is blood or mucus in the stool
- If the child is immunocompromised
- If there is a recent history of antibiotic use or stay in hospital

A3.

Antibiotics are to be considered when:

- If the child has recently returned from abroad
- If an organism causing the diarrhoea is found in the stool
- Those aged less than six months and who have Salmonella as a cause of gastroenteritis
- Those who are malnourished or immunocompromised and have Salmonella gastroenteritis
- When the following has been diagnosed:
  - *Clostridium difficile*-associated pseudomembranous enterocolitis
  - Giardiasis
  - Dysenteric shigellosis
  - Dysenteric amoebiasis
  - Cholera

Most cases of gastroenteritis are caused by a viral enteric pathogen. The illness is usually self-limiting, even when due to a bacterial or a protozoal infection. Hence antibiotic therapy is not required in most cases, with rehydration being the mainstay of treatment. The presence of dysenteric symptoms including fever, blood, or mucus in the stool, and tenesmus, may indicate the need for antibiotic therapy.

Further Reading

Guarino A, Ashkenazi S, Gendrel D, Lo Vecchio A, Shamir R, Szajewska H; et al. European Society for Pediatric Gastroenterology, Hepatology, and Nutrition/European Society for Pediatric Infectious Diseases evidence-based guidelines for the management of acute gastroenteritis in children in Europe: update 2014. *Journal of Paediatric Gastroenterology*. 2014;59:1332–152.

NICE. *Diarrhoea and Vomiting Caused by Gastroenteritis in Under 5s: Diagnosis and Management CG84*. 2014. Available from: https://www.nice.org.uk/guidance/cg84

SAQ 8 **Intussusception**

An 18-month old boy is brought in by his mother with intermittent abdominal pain and some blood in the nappies. He looks clinically unwell but his observations are normal. His abdominal X-ray is shown in Fig 18.2.

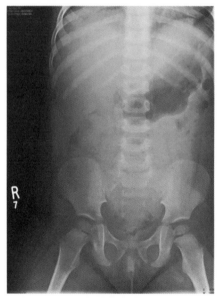

Fig.18.2 Reproduced with permission from Gardiner, R., Eisen, S. and Murphy, C. (2009). *Training in Paediatrics.* Oxford University Press. © Oxford University Press 2009. Reproduced with permission of the licensor via PLSClear.

Q1. What is the likely diagnosis?
Q2. What is the investigation of choice to confirm the diagnosis?
Q3. What are the potential complications associated with delayed diagnosis?

Answers

A1.

The likely diagnosis is intussusception, which is characterized by the triad of intermittent abdominal pain, vomiting, and a right upper quadrant mass, in association with rectal bleeding.

A2.

Ultrasound is the diagnostic modality of choice. Sensitivity and specificity have been reported to be up to 100% in the hands of expert radiologists. The classical sign to be looking for on ultrasound is the 'target sign', produced by concentric and alternating echogenic and hypoechoic bands. The plain X-ray is less specific or sensitive, but findings to look for are small bowel obstruction, an obscured liver margin and lack of air in the caecum (as in this X-ray)

A3.

Delayed recognition of intussusception may lead to:

- Bowel ischaemia and necrosis leading to perforation
- Peritonitis
- Sepsis

SAQ 9 **Acute Stridor**

A two-year-old boy presents with pyrexia, a harsh cough, and stridor.

Q1. List four causes of acute stridor in a child.
Q2. List five aspects of the Westley Croup Score that would suggest this child is safe for discharge.
Q3. List treatments including dose and route to manage a child with severe croup.

Answers

A1.

Causes of acute stridor in children include:

- Croup (acute laryngotracheobronchitis)
- Anaphylaxis
- Toxic gas inhalation
- Acute epiglottitis (high fever, sore throat, dysphagia, stridor, drooling of saliva; typically affecting children aged 2–6 years)
- Inhaled foreign body (history of a choking episode followed by stridor)
- Retropharyngeal or tonsillar abscess (fever, pain, and swelling in the neck, dysphagia, drooling of saliva, trismus, restricted neck movement)
- Bacterial tracheitis

Stridor is a sign of partial upper airway obstruction. Inspiratory stridor indicates supraglottic obstruction (extrathoracic), expiratory stridor indicates subglottic obstruction (intrathoracic), and biphasic stridor is associated with either a glottic or a subglottic lesion (intra- or extrathoracic).

A2.

Elements of the Westley croup score allowing for safe discharge include:

- No chest wall retraction
- No stridor
- No cyanosis
- Normal level of consciousness
- Good air entry

A3.

The treatment options for croup are:

- Dexamethasone 0.15 mg/kg oral single dose for mild to moderate disease, characterized by stridor at rest
- Adrenaline 5 ml (diluted with normal saline) of 1: 1000 nebulized with oxygen; repeat after 10 minutes if needed; effect lasts 2–3 hours

Further Reading

Westley CR, Cotton EK, Brooks JG. Nebulized racemic epinephrine by IPPB for the treatment of croup: a double-blind study. *American Journal of Diseases of Childhood*. 1978;132(5):484–7.

SAQ 10 **Henoch–Schönlein Purpura**

A generally unwell 5-year-old boy presents with abdominal pain and a palpable purpuric rash.

Q1. What is the likely diagnosis, and list one other differential?
Q2. The parents ask if he needs to be admitted. What assessments would help make that decision?
Q3. You decide he can be safely discharged. What management advice would you give the parents?

Answers

A1.

The likely diagnosis is Henoch–Schönlein purpura (HSP), and there is the need to exclude idiopathic thrombocytopenic purpura. HSP may present with the classical triad of purpura, arthralgia, and abdominal pain. Erythematous macules or urticaria coalesce, leading to ecchymotic lesions and palpable purpura. These are often located on the buttocks and gravity-dependent areas (lower limbs) in ambulatory children. Migratory oligoarthritis or arthralgia involves one to two large joints, usually in the lower limbs. Abdominal presentations include colicky abdominal pain, the presence of occult or gross blood in stools, and small bowel obstruction related to intussusception. Renal involvement may be associated with microscopic haematuria, and glomerulonephritis.

A2.

Initial assessments include:

- Urine dipstick—proteinuria or haematuria
- Blood pressure—hypertension
- Electrolytes and creatinine—kidney injury

A3.

Discharge advice relates to:

- Provision of analgesia (usually regular paracetamol) and bed rest
- Monitoring of early morning urine dipstick by the general practitioner
- Monitoring of blood pressure
- Return if systemically unwell or if unsure or any concerns

HSP is usually self-limiting, with resolution of symptoms within four to six weeks in most cases. Monitoring is required for early identification of renal involvement, as indicated by hypertension, macroscopic haematuria, persistent proteinuria, or the development of acute nephritic or nephrotic syndromes.

Further Reading

McCarthy HJ, Tizard EJ. Clinical practice: diagnosis and management of Henoch–Schönlein purpura. *European Journal of Paediatrics*. 2010;169:643–50.

SAQ 11 **Seizure**

You are called to the resuscitation room where you are presented with a two-year-old child with a generalized seizure.

Q1. List four important aspects of the history you would specifically ask about.
Q2. You are told that the initial seizure self-terminated within 5 minutes, but the child begins to seize again and continues to seize beyond 5 minutes. Give two treatment options including dose and route.
Q3. You decide to gain intraosseous access. Describe a site you would choose, and a contraindication.

Answers

A1.

Elements of history that are essential with this presentation include:

- Duration of the seizure
- Recent head injury
- Nature of seizure: focal or generalized
- Recent fever
- Immunosuppression
- Bleeding disorder

A2.

Initial treatment options include:

- Rectal diazepam 0.5 mg/kg
- Buccal midazolam 0.5 mg/kg
- Intravenous lorazepam 0.1 mg/kg

A3.

The preferred sites of intraosseous needle insertion include either the proximal tibia or proximal humerus (older child).
  Contraindications include:

- Osteogenesis imperfecta (if using a Cook needle)
- Osteoporosis (if using a Cook needle)
- Clotting disorders
- Fractures in the target bone

- Previous orthopaedic surgery near the insertion site
- Previous intraosseous needle insertion in the target bone within the preceding 48 hours
- Infection at the insertion site
- Loss of skin integrity

Further Reading

NICE. *Epilepsies: Diagnosis and Management CG137.* 2018. Available from: https://www.nice.org.uk/guidance/cg137

SAQ 12 **Chicken Pox**

A fully vaccinated two-year-old is brought to the emergency department. He has been off his food for a few days and has been quite 'clingy'. His mother noticed a few red marks appearing on his belly last night but did the 'glass test' which was negative, so she wasn't too worried. This morning however he was covered head to toe in red spots, so she thought she'd better get him checked. His rash is shown in Fig. 18.3.

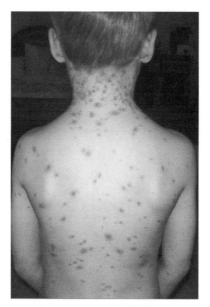

Fig. 18.3 Reproduced with permission from Lewis-Jones, S. (2010). *Paediatric Dermatology*. Oxford University Press. © Oxford University Press, 2010. Reproduced with permission of the licensor via PLSClear.

Q1. What is the most likely diagnosis?
Q2. Name three possible complications.
Q3. The mother asks if it is contagious. What is your advice?

Answers

A1.

The most likely diagnosis is chicken pox (varicella) caused by the varicella-zoster virus. In children, in whom it is a benign and self-limited illness, there is usually no prodrome or a mild prodrome of fever, malaise, anorexia, and pharyngitis. Prodromal symptoms are often seen in adolescents and adults. Crops of erythematous macules on the head, face, trunk, and proximal limbs progress centripetally over 12–24 hours to papules, vesicles, or bullae (surrounded by an erythematous halo, with a dewdrop on a rose petal appearance), pustules, and crusting. Crusts detach leaving areas of temporary hypopigmentation. Lesions are seen in all stages of progression simultaneously.

A2.

Complications of chickenpox include:

- Secondary bacterial infections caused by Group A streptococcus, leading to impetigo, cellulitis, and erysipelas. Bacterial superinfection can lead to sepsis and septic shock
- Pneumonia, which can be viral or secondary bacterial
- Central nervous system complications: encephalitis; Guillain–Barré syndrome; Reye syndrome; acute cerebellar ataxia
- Haemorrhagic complications: thrombocytopenia, purpura
- Disseminated varicella, in immunocompromised patients

All these are more likely if the subject is immunocompromised.

A3.

Chickenpox is highly contagious. The virus is transmissible 1–2 days before the rash appears and then until all the vesicles have crusted over. After exposure it takes around 2 weeks to become symptomatic. If vaccinated a person can still carry the virus and although one episode usually confers lifetime immunity, this is not always the case.

Further Reading

RCOG. *Chickenpox in Pregnancy. Green-top Guideline No 13.* 2015. Available from: https://www.rcog.org.uk/en/guidelines-research-services/guidelines/gtg13/

SAQ 13 **Kawasaki Disease**

You are evaluating a four-year-old girl with a seven-day history of persistent fever, which is not responding to antibiotics prescribed by her general practitioner. You wonder if she may have Kawasaki disease.

Q1. What features. other than fever, help arrive at a diagnosis of Kawasaki disease? List four
Q2. What initial treatments may be recommended? List two.
Q3. Name a complication that early treatment may prevent.

Answers

A1.

Kawasaki disease is an acute multisystem vasculitis of childhood, of unknown aetiology, and is diagnosed based on its clinical presentation, which includes:

- Fever of at least 38.5°C for at least 5 days; typically, unresponsive to antipyretics and antibiotics
- Four of the following five abnormalities:
  - Conjunctival injection (non-purulent; bilateral; primarily bulbar conjunctiva, with sparing of the corneoscleral limbus)
  - Oral mucosal changes (red, swollen, and cracked lips; strawberry tongue; no discrete oral lesions or exudates)
  - Cervical lymphadenopathy, often unilateral and large (>1.5 cm in diameter), with mild or no overlying erythema, and not fluctuant
  - Rash (may be maculopapular or polymorphic erythema, but not petechial, bullous, or vesicular)
  - Swollen red hands and feet (erythema or indurative oedema and later, in the second week of illness, membranous desquamation starting around the nail bed)

A2.

Initial treatment may include:

- Single infusion of intravenous polyclonal immunoglobulin 2 g/kg over 8–12 hours; given 5–10 days after the onset of fever
- High dose aspirin 30–50 mg/kg/day (in four divided doses) until the child is afebrile and C-reactive protein (CRP) normal and 3–5 mg/kg/day thereafter until a normal echocardiogram is seen at 6 weeks after the onset of symptoms

A3.

Early treatment may prevent the development of giant coronary artery aneurysms. Early treatment with intravenous immunoglobulin reduces the incidence of aneurysms, which can be recognized by echocardiography.

Further Reading

McCrindle BW, Rowley AH, Newburger JW, Burns JC, Bolger AF, Gewitz M, et al. Diagnosis, treatment, and long-term management of Kawasaki Disease: a scientific statement for health professionals from the American Heart Association. *Circulation*. 2017;135:e1–e73.

SAQ 14 **Neonatology**

Six-day-old baby Justin has been brought in by his mother to the emergency department. He has not been feeding well for the last 24 hours and goes blue when he takes a bottle.

Q1. List six signs of respiratory distress in a neonate.
Q2. List six causes of respiratory distress in the neonatal period.
Q3. Justin is tachycardic at 160, with a delayed capillary refill. He has bibasal crackles on auscultation of the lungs and a palpable liver edge on abdominal palpation. What is the likely diagnosis and how would you manage him?

Answers

A1.

Signs of neonatal respiratory distress include:

- Tachypnoea (respiratory rate >60/minute)
- Intercostal and subcostal recession—accessory muscle use
- Flaring of alae nasi—accessory muscle use
- Grunting—forced expiration against closed glottis
- Cyanosis—>5 g/L of desaturated haemoglobin
- Apnoea
- Tracheal tug—accessory muscles

A2.

Potential causes of neonatal respiratory distress can be classified as:

- Upper airway
  - i. Laryngomalacia
- Lower airway
  - i. Infant respiratory distress syndrome (hyaline membrane disease)
  - ii. Congenital pneumonia
  - iii. Meconium aspiration
  - iv. Transient tachypnoea of the newborn
  - v. Pneumothorax
- Cardiac
  - i. Heart failure
  - ii. Myocarditis
  - iii. Pericardial effusion
  - iv. Congenital heart disease—ventricular septal defect, duct-dependant lesions; transposition of the great vessels
- Structural
  - i. Congenital diaphragmatic hernia
  - ii. Congenital cystic lesions

- Anaemia
- Infection
- Metabolic causes

A3.

A duct-dependent lesion such as hypoplastic left heart, critical aortic stenosis, coarctation of the aorta is likely. Initial management includes:

- Close observation in the emergency department
- Chest X-ray
- Full septic screen
- A cardiac shadow greater than 0% of transthoracic diameter is indicative of cardiac disease
- Arterial blood gases
- Cautious fluid therapy
- Prostaglandin E2 infusion
- Discussion with CATS (children's acute transport service)/tertiary paediatric unit

SAQ 15 **Bronchiolitis**

An anxious mother brings her six-month-old male infant to the emergency department as he appears to be coughing, breathing fast, and sounds 'wheezy'. You make a diagnosis of acute bronchiolitis based on your clinical assessment.

Q1. List three clinical signs suggestive of bronchiolitis.
Q2. List four factors in determining the severity of the presentation.
Q3. You have decided to send the child home. List three specific forms of advice you would give the mother.

Answers

A1.

The diagnosis of bronchiolitis is suggested by the presence of:

- Tachypnoea
- Chest recession, which may be subcostal, intercostal, and supraclavicular
- Bilateral fine inspiratory crackles and/or bilateral high-pitched expiratory wheeze on auscultation

Bronchiolitis mainly affects children under two years of age and is most common in the first year of life, with peak incidence between 3 and 6 months of age. There is typically a prodromal upper respiratory tract infection lasting 1 to 3 days. Peak prevalence is in the winter months (November to March).

A2.

Factors associated with increased severity in bronchiolitis include:

- Poor feeding (<50% usual fluid intake in the preceding 24 hours)
- A history of apnoeic episodes
- Cyanosis
- Lethargy
- Persistent oxygen saturation of 92% or less, despite oxygen therapy
- Inadequate oral intake
- Persistent severe respiratory distress, including severe tachypnoea (>70 breaths per minute), marked chest recession, and grunting
- High risk patients, such as age under 3 months, premature birth (especially under 32 weeks), chronic lung disease of prematurity, haemodynamically significant congenital heart disease, neuromuscular disorders, and immunodeficiency

A3.

Most infants with acute bronchiolitis have mild disease and can be managed at home with primary care support. The mother should be given the following information, preferably with an accompanying written advice sheet:

- The importance of maintaining adequate hydration
- Red flag symptoms indicating deterioration and warranting medical attention: apnoea or cyanosis, reduced feeding, reduced urine output (wet nappies), worsening work of breathing (nasal flaring, grunting, drowsiness)
- Avoidance of smoking at home
- There is no need for antibiotics or other prescribed medication, as the illness is viral and usually self-limiting

Further Reading

NICE. *Bronchiolitis in Children: Diagnosis and Management NG9.* 2015. Available from: https://www.nice.org.uk/guidance/ng9

SAQ 16 **Febrile Convulsion**

A two-year-old female child is brought to the resuscitation room following a witnessed generalized seizure at home. The seizure stopped spontaneously before the ambulance personnel arrived. On questioning her mother, it becomes clear that the child has felt 'hot' over the past 24 hours. The child is otherwise well, and nothing like this has happened before.

Q1. List four characteristics of a simple febrile seizure.

Q2. What makes a febrile seizure complex? List three features.

Q3. You are discharging a child home after a simple febrile seizure, with no underlying worrying diagnosis. Give three elements of advice you would give the parents if another seizure were to occur.

Answers

A1.

A simple febrile seizure has the following characteristics:

- The age of the child is between 6 months and 5 years; the majority occur in children between 12 and 18 months of age, and on the first day of onset of fever.
- The seizure is generalized and lasts less than 15 minutes; usually last between 1 to 5 minutes.
- The seizure type is either generalized clonic or generalized tonic-clonic.
- The seizure occurs only once during a 24-hour period.
- The child does not have any neurological abnormality on examination or based on developmental history.

A2.

A complex febrile seizure is characterized by:

- Focal features during the seizure, such as temporary limb weakness
- Prolonged, more than 15 minutes
- Recurrent seizures in the same episode of illness
- Incomplete recovery after one hour

A3.

Advice if a further seizure occurs includes:

- Protect from injury
- Do not restrain or put anything in the mouth of the child
- Time the seizure

- Place in the recovery position on a protected surface after the seizure stops, after checking the airway
- Dial 99 and call an ambulance if the seizure lasts more than 5 minutes

Further Reading

Patel N, Ram D, Swiderska N, Mewasingh LD, Newton RW, Offringa M. Febrile seizures. *British Medical Journal*. 2015;351:h4240.

SAQ 17 **Non-accidental Injury**

You are preparing a talk on the recognition of non-accidental injury in children as part of a teaching session for the FY2 trainees in your department. In this connection, you must provide some key pieces of information for your audience.

Q1. List four patterns of fracture, based on anatomical site, which suggest non-accidental injury.
Q2. What are the features of shaken baby syndrome? List three.
Q3. What types of bruises are more likely to inflicted? List three.

Answers

A1.

Some patterns and locations of fracture suggest non-accidental injury, including:

- Metaphyseal, bucket handle, or corner fractures of long bones, which indicate torsional or shearing stress on the bone
- Posterior rib fractures, which result from antero-posterior compression as in forcible squeezing
- Fractures of the lateral end of the clavicles
- Fractures of the scapula
- Fractures of the sternum
- Fractures of the spinous processes of vertebrae
- Multiple fractures at different stages of healing, in the absence of a medical condition predisposing to fragile bones
- Fractures of long bones in preambulatory children
- Complex skull fractures, including multiple, bilateral, diastatic, or those that cross suture lines

A2.

The shaken baby syndrome is a form of abusive head trauma caused by the violent shaking of an infant or young child (usually up to the age of 5 years) by the shoulders, arms, or legs, and is characterized by a triad of:

- Subdural haemorrhage, caused by the rupture of bridging veins connecting the dura to the pia-arachnoid, which can be multiple and may be accompanied by subarachnoid haemorrhage
- Unilateral or bilateral retinal haemorrhages
- Encephalopathy

There is usually no external evidence of head injury. There is some current controversy about the causative mechanism of this injury.

A3.

Bruises that are inflicted may show the following characteristics:

- Bruising in children who are not independently mobile
- Bruising in babies
- Bruises away from bony prominences, such as on the buttocks, thighs, abdomen, cheeks, eyes, ears, neck, axillae, and genitalia
- Multiple bruises in clusters
- Multiple bruises of uniform shape and size
- Patterned bruises carrying the imprint of an implement (such as linear objects causing tramline bruising, as with belt buckles, rods, or sticks), of the hand (from slapping), of fingertips, or of a cord or rope causing curvilinear loop marks
- Bruises with surrounding petechiae

Bruising in ambulatory children is common, but is very unusual in children who have not commenced crawling (i.e. with no independent mobility). Accidental bruising is usually over bony prominences, as in the shins, knees, elbows, and forehead.

Further Reading

NICE. *Child* Abuse and Neglect. NG 76, 2017 Available from: https://www.nice.org.uk/guidance/ng76

Chapter 19 **Respiratory Medicine**

SAQ 1 **Community-acquired Pneumonia**

You see a 54-year-old man in the emergency department. He saw his general practitioner a few days earlier as he had symptoms of a lower respiratory tract infection. He is unhappy that he was not prescribed antibiotics.

Q1. What is the National Institute for Health and Care Excellence (NICE) guidance on antibiotic prescription in patients with lower respiratory tract infection symptoms for a C-reactive protein (CRP) level of 17?

Q2. You decide, based on clinical, biochemical, and radiological findings today that he probably should be started on antibiotics for community-acquired pneumonia. How long should he expect to wait before his cough has reduced?

Q3. In moderate to severe community-acquired pneumonia what would be the antibiotic duration?

Answers

A1.

If a point-of-care test for CRP is available, then the following results can guide antibiotic treatment:

- Most people do not need antibiotics if the CRP is less than 20 mg/L
- If CRP is between 20 mg/L and 100 mg/L, it is advisable to consider a delayed prescription for antibiotics
- If CRP is over 100 mg/L, then antibiotics are recommended

A2.

Cough may last for approximately six weeks. With respect to other symptoms:

- 1 week: fever should have resolved
- 4 weeks: chest pain and sputum production should have substantially reduced
- 6 weeks: breathlessness should have substantially reduced
- 3 months: most symptoms should have resolved but fatigue may still be present
- 6 months: most people will feel back to normal

A3.

Antibiotics are usually prescribed for 7–10 days. It is advisable to use dual therapy using amoxicillin and a macrolide in moderate cases and beta-lactamase stable beta lactam and a macrolide for severe cases.

Further Reading

NICE. *Pneumonia in Adults: Diagnosis and Management CG191*. 2014. Available from: https://www.nice.org.uk/guidance/cg191

SAQ 2 **Pneumonia**

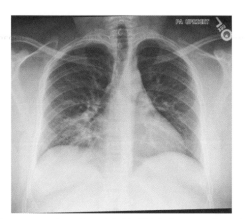

Fig. 19.1 Reproduced with permission from Abujudeh, H. (2016). *Emergency Radiology*. Oxford University Press USA. © Oxford University Press 2016. Reproduced with permission of the licensor via PLSClear.

Fig. 19.1 shows the radiograph of a 77-year-old man who presents with fever and a productive cough.

Q1. What are the radiological findings?

Q2. Describe a clinical scoring system relevant to this patient's presentation.

Q3. List three common bacterial causative organisms.

Answers

A1.

This X-ray demonstrates right middle lobe consolidation, with loss of contour of the right heart border.

A2.

CURB 65 is a relevant clinical scoring system for community-acquired pneumonia. The components of CURB 65 are outlined in Table 19.1.

Table 19.1

Confusion	New AMTS <8	+1
Urea (BUN)	Urea >7	+1
Respiratory rate	RR >30	+1
Blood pressure	Systolic <90	+1

Reproduced from *Thorax*, Lim, W.S. et al. Defining community acquired pneumonia severity on presentation to hospital: an international derivation and validation study. 2003; 58:377–82. http://dx.doi.org/10.1136/thorax.58.5.377. Copyright © 2003, BMJ Publishing Group Ltd and the British Thoracic Society. With permission from BMJ Publishing Group Ltd.

A3.

Bacterial organisms causing community-acquired pneumonia include the following:

Streptococcus pneumoniae, Haemophilus influenza, Mycoplasma pneumoniae, Moraxella catarrhalis, Legionella pneumophila.

Further Reading

Lims WS, van der Eerden MM, Laing R, Boersma WG, Karalus N, Town GI, et al. Defining community-acquired pneumonia severity on presentation to hospital: an international derivation and validation study *Thorax*. 2003;58:377–82.

SAQ 3 **Non-invasive Ventilation**

A 51-year-old gentleman, who has been a lifelong heavy cigarette smoker, presents to your emergency department with progressively worsening cough and shortness of breath. On arrival, he is unable to talk in full sentences, is dyspnoeic with a respiratory rate of 24/minute, and his oxygen saturation is 82% on room air. There is widespread quiet expiratory wheeze on auscultation. Your working diagnosis is that of an acute infective exacerbation of chronic obstructive pulmonary disease. You analyse an arterial blood gas sample, and the result is as follows:

pH 7.22 pO_2 7.9 pCO_2 8.8 HCO_3 34.

Q1. Given the most likely diagnosis, outline your initial management of this gentleman. List four key interventions.

Q2. What are the indications for non-invasive ventilation? List four.

Q3. Explain how non-invasive ventilation is beneficial in terms of respiratory physiology.

Answers

A1.

Management of an acute exacerbation of chronic obstructive pulmonary disease (COPD) consists of:

- Supplemental oxygen to maintain arterial oxygen saturations of 88 to 92%. This may be controlled oxygen therapy using a 24% or 28% Venturi mask, or nasal cannulae with a flow rate of 1–2 litres a minute
- Nebulized salbutamol 5 mg repeated/back to back
- Nebulized ipratropium 500 micrograms
- Intravenous access and blood tests (full blood count, urea and electrolytes, BNP)
- Antibiotics, such as amoxicillin, co-amoxiclav, tetracycline
- Corticosteroid, either prednisolone 40 mg oral or hydrocortisone 200 mg intravenous
- Bedside investigations: chest X-ray, 12-lead electrocardiogram (ECG), repeat arterial blood gas

An acute exacerbation of COPD is defined as a sustained worsening of the patient's condition from the stable state and beyond the normal day-to-day variation, which is acute in onset and can be associated with worsening breathlessness, increased sputum volume, changing sputum colour, and cough.

A2.

Indications for non-invasive ventilation (NIV) include:

- Obstructive sleep apnoea
- Acute cardiogenic pulmonary oedema
- Acute hypercapnic COPD with respiratory acidosis (type 2 respiratory failure)
- Chest wall/neuromuscular disease
- Ceiling of treatment in patients not suitable for intermittent positive pressure ventilation

A3.

Effects of NIV on the respiratory system include:

- Increases oxygenation
- Provides PEEP (positive end-expiratory pressure) and splints open alveoli at the end of expiration. Opens up atelectatic and fluid-filled lung. Recruits more of the alveoli for gas exchange
- Reduces the work of breathing
- Increases functional residual capacity
- Drives alveolar fluid back into the circulation

Further Reading

BTS/ICS Guidelines for the ventilatory management of acute hypercapnic respiratory failure in adults. Thorax, 2016, 71: Supplement 2

SAQ 4 **Capnography**

Q1. According to the European Resuscitation Council guidelines, capnography should be used in adults and children to provide information on which four aspects of resuscitation?

Q2. What are the three determinants of end tidal carbon dioxide?

Q3. Is a higher or lower end tidal carbon dioxide prognostic of ROSC (return of spontaneous circulation) and discharge from hospital following cardio-pulmonary resuscitation?

Answers

A1.

Capnography provides information on:

- Quality of chest compressions
- Return of spontaneous circulation
- Tracheal tube placement
- Normoventilation

A2.

The three determinants of end tidal carbon dioxide are:

- Carbon dioxide produced by cellular metabolism
- Carbon dioxide transport to the lungs (i.e. cardiac output)
- Carbon dioxide elimination by ventilation

A3.

A higher end tidal carbon dioxide is predictive of ROSC and potential discharge from hospital. Some studies have shown that below a certain threshold of end tidal carbon dioxide (1.3 kpa) non-survival is almost guaranteed.

Further Reading

Mohr NM, Stoltze A, Ahmed A, Kiscaden E, Shane D. Using continuous quantitative capnography for emergency department procedural sedation: a systematic review and cost-effectiveness analysis *Internal and Emergency Medicine*. 2018;13(1):75–85.

SAQ 5 **Asthma**

A 28-year-old female with a history of asthma is brought to the resuscitation room with acute shortness of breath. On arrival, she cannot speak in complete sentences. Her vital signs are: HR 110, RR 30, BP 127/81, SpO$_2$ 92% (on air), and peak expiratory flow rate (PEFR) 200 (normally 500).

Q1. What is the severity of her asthma at presentation?
Q2. What are the features of a life-threatening attack? List five.
Q3. Other than high-flow oxygen, what treatments would you institute to optimize her initial medical management?

Answers

A1.

This is a severe attack (tachycardia, tachypnoea, PEFR 30–50%, inability to complete sentences).

A2.

Life-threatening features of acute asthma are:

- Unable to talk
- Exhaustion
- Confusion
- Cyanosis of lips and tongue on room air
- Silent chest
- Saturation <90%
- PFR <33% of predicted or best
- No response to beta 2 agonist therapy
- Bradycardia
- Coma
- Hypotension

A3.

Treatments that should be initiated on arrival include the following:

- Nebulized salbutamol
- Nebulized ipratropium
- Corticosteroid (40 mg prednisolone orally or 200 mg hydrocortisone intravenous)
- Intravenous magnesium (2 g intravenous over 20 mins)

If not responding, other measures to consider include:

- Intravenous. salbutamol 250 mcg bolus then 5–10 mcg/minute
- Intravenous aminophylline 250 mg loading dose, then infusion of 0.5 mg/kg/h
- Intravenous ketamine 0.75 mg/kg

Further Reading

BTS/SIGN. British Guideline for the Management of Asthma, SIGN 153. 2016. Available from: https://www.sign.ac.uk/sign-153-british-guideline-on-the-management-of-asthma.html

SAQ 6 **Chronic Obstructive Pulmonary Disease**

A 75-year-old man with acute shortness of breath is brought to the emergency department by ambulance. The ambulance technician started him on 60% oxygen prior to arrival in hospital. He is now unable to speak and no other history is available. On examination, he has nicotine stained fingers. His pulse rate is 120 beats per minute and respiratory rate 32 breaths per minute. His barrel shaped chest revealed occasional scattered wheezing. A chest X-ray shows overinflated lungs but no pneumothorax.

The arterial blood gas report, with the patient on 60% room air, is as follows:

PaO_2	7.1 kpa
PH	7.17
$PaCO_2$	9.4 kpa
Base excess	−10 mmol/L

Q1. Describe the abnormalities on arterial blood gas analysis.
Q2. What is your diagnosis?
Q3. What would be your immediate action?

Answers

A1.

The arterial blood gas reveals severe hypoxia, not corrected by oxygen therapy, and combined respiratory and metabolic acidosis.

A2.

The diagnosis is acute exacerbation of COPD with type 2 respiratory failure.

A3.

The immediate actions include reducing the inspired oxygen concentration to 24%, commencement of nebulized salbutamol nebulizers and administration of steroids. Then recheck arterial blood gases after 30 minutes.

Further Reading

NICE. *Chronic Obstructive Pulmonary Disease in Over 16s: Diagnosis and Management* NG115, 2018

SAQ 7 **Chronic Obstructive Pulmonary Disease 2**

A 55-year-old man, who has been a lifelong smoker, is brought is brought in by the ambulance service to your resuscitation room with acute shortness of breath. His pulse rate is 118/minute and respiratory rate 34 breaths/min. He has widespread expiratory wheeze on examination.

Q1. Name five differential diagnoses in this patient.
Q2. What are the indications for ventilation of this patient?
Q3 What are the indications for admission to hospital? List four.

Answers

A1.

The differential diagnoses for this presentation include:

- Pneumonia—viral or bacterial
- Spontaneous pneumothorax
- Pulmonary embolism
- Myocardial infarction with acute pulmonary oedema
- Acute asthma
- Respiratory muscle diseases such as poliomyelitis, myasthenia gravis, Guillain–Barré syndrome, motor neurone disease
- Brain stem disorders
- Sedative drugs

A2.

The indications for assisted ventilation are:

- Persistent hypercapnic ventilatory failure despite optimal medical therapy (controlled oxygen, nebulizers, steroids, antibiotics)
- PH <7.35
- Arterial pCO_2 >6 kPa

A3.

The indications for admission include:

- Inability to cope at home
- Severe presentation
- Cyanotic
- On home oxygen
- Delirium

- Significant comorbidity
- Changes on chest X-ray
- pH <7.35
- pO_2 <7

Further Reading

Global Initiative for Obstructive Lung Disease. *Guidelines*. 2017. Available from: https://goldcopd.org/wp-content/uploads/2016/12/wms-GOLD-2017-Pocket-Guide.pdf

SAQ 8 Massive Haemoptysis

A 60-year-old male, known to have cancer of the right lung, is brought to the resuscitation room with ongoing haemoptysis and an estimated blood loss of around 500 ml. On initial assessment, his vital signs are: heart rate 110/minute, respiratory rate 24/minute, blood pressure 90/60 mm Hg, and SpO$_2$ on room air 90%.

Q1. List three immediate priorities for management
Q2. What definitive management is required in the resuscitation room?
Q3. How can the bleeding be controlled?

Answers

A1.

In the presence of massive haemoptysis, the following are indicated:

- Nurse with affected side down (in lateral decubitus) to protect the unaffected lung
- High-flow oxygen
- Restoration of circulating blood volume: venous access and commencement of infusion of packed red cells (crystalloid only if blood not available)—consider declaring massive haemorrhage

A2.

Early control of the airway with tracheal tube placement, is indicated.

A3.

Control of the bleeding requires localization and treatment of the source via either flexible fibreoptic or rigid bronchoscopy.
   Other measures may include:

- Tranexamic acid 1 g intravenous
- Vitamin K 5 mg intravenous
- Prothrombin complex concentrate, for example, Octaplex® 50 u/kg (if on warfarin)

SAQ 9 **Spontaneous Pneumothorax**

A 35-year-old non-smoker presents with sudden onset of shortness of breath. The X-ray is shown in Fig 19.2:

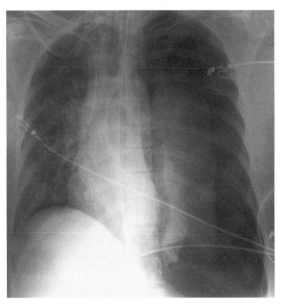

Fig. 19.2 Reproduced with permission from Seiden, D. and Corbett, S. (2013). *Lachman's Case Studies in Anatomy.* 5th ed. Oxford University Press USA. © Oxford University Press 2013. Reproduced with permission of the licensor via PLSClear.

Q1. What is the diagnosis?
Q2. What is the initial treatment, and describe the landmarks?
Q3. What is the definitive treatment?

Answers

A1.

The chest X-ray shows a left-sided tension pneumothorax with deviation of the mediastinal structures to the right.

A2.

If tension is suspected, the traditional teaching suggests a needle decompression in the mid-cla-vicular line in the second intercostal space. The tension may also be decompressed just anterior to the mid-axillary line in the fourth to sixth intercostal spaces. The British Thoracic Society guideline recommends aspiration of a primary pneumothorax as first management if the size is bigger than 2 cm as measured at the hilum.

A3.

The definitive treatment involves chest drain placement (tube thoracostomy) employing Seldinger technique, size 12–14 Fr, in the triangle of safety: posterior to lateral border of pectoralis major and anterior to latissimus dorsi, above the fifth intercostal space.

Further Reading

British Thoracic Society. *Pleural Disease Guidelines*. Available from: https://www.brit-thoracic.org.uk/search/?query=pleural+disease+guidelines

SAQ 10 **Subcutaneous Emphysema of Chest Wall**

A 78-year-old gentleman attends after a fall and presents with chest pain. The X-ray is shown in Fig. 19.3.

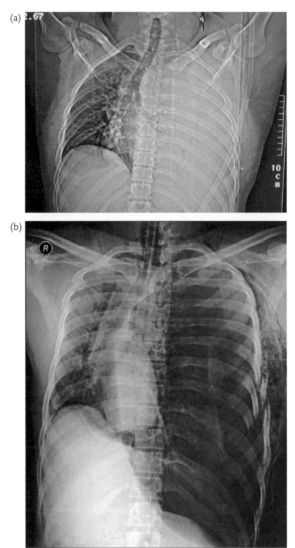

Fig. 19.3 Reproduced with permission from Spoors, C. and Kiff, K. (2010). *Training in Anaesthesia*. Oxford University Press. © Oxford University Press 2010. Reproduced with permission of the licensor via PLSClear.

Q1. Describe the chest X-ray.
Q2. What do the chest X-ray findings suggest?
Q3. What would be your management?

Answers

A1.

The chest X-ray shows surgical (or subcutaneous) emphysema on the left lateral chest wall, with pockets of air in the soft tissue planes.

A2.

This appearance suggests a likely rib fracture with pneumothorax (unless there is an open wound on the left chest wall, which could be a theoretical cause of subcutaneous emphysema).

A3.

The free air usually does not need any specific treatment, but its presence should warrant consideration of underlying significant causative injuries. High-resolution computed tomography (CT) chest with contrast may be indicated for further investigation. Severe surgical emphysema may cause upper airway and jugular vein compression, with airway and cardiovascular compromise, with tracking of air into the neck. Air may also track into the mediastinum, retroperitoneum, scrotum, and lower limbs. If very tense and symptomatic, releasing skin incisions may be needed.

SAQ 11 **Asthma 2**

A 24-year-old asthmatic man is brought to the emergency department complaining of severe short-ness of breath. He is having difficulty speaking. You immediately commence him on a salbutamol nebulizer, run on high-flow oxygen, and take a blood gas sample.

Blood gas report: patient on high-flow oxygen

PaO_2	12.1 kpa
PH	7.30
$PaCO_2$	6.0 kpa
Base excess	−7 mmol/L

Q1. Describe the abnormalities on arterial blood gas analysis.
Q2. Are these findings consistent with a severe asthma attack?
Q3. How would you treat this patient if he did not improve and what are the indications for ventilation of this patient?

Answers

A1.

Arterial blood gas analysis shows severe hypoxaemia with metabolic acidosis.

A2.

Yes. This result is typical of an asthmatic beginning to develop type 2 respiratory failure with failure of ventilation.

A3.

Ongoing management includes:

- Continue high-flow oxygen
- Call for expert help
- Repeat 5 mg salbutamol nebulizers
- Add ipratropium bromide 0.5 mg nebulized for 15 mins
- Add prednisolone 40–50 mg orally or intravenous hydrocortisone 200 mg
- Consider continuous salbutamol nebulizers 5–10 mg/hour
- Consider intravenous magnesium sulfate 2 g over 20 minutes
- Correct fluid/electrolytes especially disturbances in potassium levels
- Chest X-ray

Intubation and ventilation are indicated when blood gases on 60% O_2 show:

- Po_2 <8 kpa
- PH <7.2
- PCO_2 >6.7

SAQ 12 **Asthma 3**

A 24-year-old obese female presents with an exacerbation of previously diagnosed asthma.

Q1. Give three features of life-threatening asthma.

Q2. Besides nebulized bronchodilators and oral or intravenous steroid therapy, what treatment does the British Thoracic Society recommend as the next management step?

Q3. What criteria would you use to decide whether to admit or discharge the patient?

Answers

A1.

Life-threatening features of asthma include:

- Arterial oxygen saturation <92%
- Silent chest/poor respiratory effort
- Cyanosis
- Bradycardia
- Hypotension

A2.

1.2–2 g of intravenous magnesium should be administered.

A3.

The peak flow helps in advising the need for hospital admission. If the PEFR after 1 hour is more than 75% of the baseline PEFR, consider discharge, unless the patient has other features mandating admission (previous near-fatal exacerbation, worsening of symptoms while on steroids, learning disability, poor compliance, or still symptomatic).

Chapter 20 **Trauma**

SAQ 1 **Fascia Iliaca Block**

An elderly lady has fallen in her nursing home, sustaining a fractured neck of femur. You decide she needs a fascia iliaca block for pain relief.

Q1. Give at least three indications for a fascia iliaca compartment block.

Q2. Label Fig. 20.1 with the femoral nerve and the fascia iliaca:

Q3. Which local anaesthetic agent will you use and at what dose?

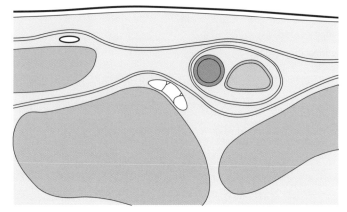

Fig. 20.1 Reproduced with permission from Warman, P., Conn, D., Nicholls, B. and Wilkinson, D. (2014). *Regional Anaesthesia, Stimulation, and Ultrasound Techniques*. Oxford University Press. © Oxford University Press 2014. Reproduced with permission of the licensor via PLSClear.

Answers

A1.

Indications for fascia iliaca block include:

- Perioperative analgesia for fractured neck/shaft of the femur
- Additional analgesia during hip surgery
- Analgesia for above-knee amputations
- Analgesia for applying plaster to children with a fractured femur
- Analgesia when combined with a sciatic nerve block for knee operations
- Analgesia to cover pain from lower leg tourniquet during awake operations

The superficial fascial layer of the iliopsoas muscle (fascia iliaca) at the anterior edge of the ilium may be identified with ultrasound or a blind technique may be employed. The needle is introduced just beneath this fascial plane. Local anaesthetic solution is then injected. In order to be effective, the block requires a high volume of anaesthetic (about 40 ml). This fluid that accumulates then redistributes beneath the fascia and eventually contacts the nerves of the lumbar plexus. The nerves that are blocked using this technique are the lateral femoral cutaneous nerve, the femoral nerve, and the obturator nerves.

A surface landmark technique is perfectly satisfactory in the absence of ultrasound. The injection point lies approximately one-third along, and one centimetre below, a line drawn from the anterior superior iliac spine (ASIS) to the pubic tubercle. Positioning the needle correctly relies on its feel as it passes first through the fascia lata and then the fascia iliaca (two pops).

A2.

Fig. 20.2 shows the femoral nerve and the fascia iliaca as follows: **1** fascia lata; **2** fascia iliaca; black arrow, lateral cutaneous nerve of the thigh; N, femoral nerve; A, femoral artery; V, femoral vein; IM, iliacus muscle; PM, pectineus muscle; SM, sartorius muscle.

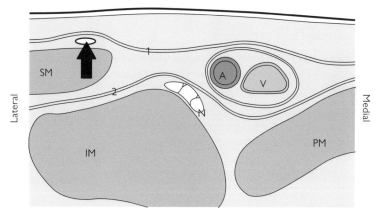

Fig. 20.2 Reproduced with permission from Warman, P., Conn, D., Nicholls, B. and Wilkinson, D. (2014). *Regional Anaesthesia, Stimulation, and Ultrasound Techniques*. Oxford University Press. © Oxford University Press 2014. Reproduced with permission of the licensor via PLSClear.

A3.

The agent of choice is bupivacaine:

- The maximum allowable dose is 2 mg/kg
- This technique employs a high-volume injection thus use 40 ml of 0.25%
  - A 0.25% solution has a concentration of 2.5 mg per ml
  - 40 ml = 100 mg

Further Reading

Dalens B, Vanneuville G, Tanguy A. Comparison of the fascia iliaca compartment block with the 3-in-1 block in children. *Anaesthesia and Analgesia*. 1989;69:705–13.

SAQ 2 **Thoracotomy**

Prompted by a recent case in the department your trainees have requested a teaching session focusing on thoracotomy in trauma in a prehospital setting, and it is your turn to teach. You do not do prehospital shifts yourself, so you do some background reading to refresh your knowledge.

Q1. What is the indication for thoracotomy in a prehospital setting?
Q2. List three of the interventions that may take place within the thoracic cavity once the chest is open.
Q3. What are the indications for emergency department thoracotomy in cases of blunt trauma?

A1.

Thoracostomy is indicated for:

- Penetrating thoracic injury with *previously* witnessed cardiac activity (i.e. signs of life)
- The general consensus is that the intervention must take place within 10 minutes following loss of these signs of life

It is stated by the standard operating procedure written for UK HEMS (Helicopter Emergency Medical Service) that the decision to perform the procedure should be made within 10–15 seconds of arriving on scene and establishing the clinical status of the patient.

A2.

Interventions within the thoracic cavity may include:

- Internal cardiac massage
- Manual or instrumental aortic clamping
- Lacerations to the myocardium may be managed initially by placing a balloon catheter into the chamber and inflating the balloon. Sutures may be placed in the myocardium
- Lung twist if bleeding is detected from around the hilum
- Internal defibrillation or finger flick to stimulate contractility
- Call for help

A3.

A 2015 *Emergency Medical Journal* meta-analysis involved:

- 1400 cases in total
- <1% survival (20 survivors)
- Survival more likely if:
  - Loss of vital signs in the emergency department (brought in with signs of life of if HEMS arrive on scene and patient has signs of life)
  - No cardiopulmonary resuscitation (CPR) (as chest compressions will exacerbate thoracic trauma, disrupt clot, impair ventilation, and compress an empty heart)
  - There is no other reason for the patient to die (e.g. catastrophic head injury)

So, in summary, it should be considered in selected cases.

Further Reading

Hunt PA, Greaves I, Owens WA. Emergency thoracotomy in thoracic trauma—a review Injury. 2006;37:1–19.

SAQ 3 **Major Trauma**

A 62-year-old building site foreman fell 3 metres from scaffolding onto some rubble. A site worker called 999 and the specialist dispatcher, working on the HEMS desk at the control centre of the London Ambulance Service, agrees to deploy the air ambulance. On arrival, the HEMS crew find him immobile in the left lateral position, with noisy breathing and Glasgow Coma Score (GCS) of 8. His pulse was 59 and irregular (known atrial fibrillation). The blood pressure is 181/101 mm Hg. There is a very large contusion with a deep laceration to the occiput. There appear to be no other injuries.

Q1. Based on the mechanism, what are the possible injuries from top to toe? List four.
Q2. Outline the overall approach to the management of this patient both prehospital and in the emergency department. List four interventions.
Q3. On arrival at the major trauma centre, the patient's core temperature is measured at 33°C. Why is temperature so important in the context of managing trauma patients and what is meant by the triad of death?

Answers

A1.

The possible injuries from top to toe include:

- Head injury: likely traumatic brain injury
- Cervical spine injury
- Chest injury—rib fractures likely with underlying haemopneumothorax or lung contusion; possible flail chest
- Abdominal injury—injury to spleen not improbable with intraperitoneal bleeding
- Pelvic injury
- Vertebral column injury from axial load. Blow our fracture which may lead to risk of spinal cord injury
- Long bone injury (e.g. closed or open fractures of lower or upper limbs)

A2.

The overall approach comprises:

- Application of a semi-rigid cervical collar (but not too tight as may raise intracranial pressure).
- Establishment of intravenous access. If not possible, then humeral head intraosseous access.
- Securing the airway based on mechanism, likely injuries, and Glasgow Coma Score. The patient needs rapid sequence induction with fentanyl, ketamine, and rocuronium. Maintain manual in-line immobilization.
- Give blood products (with fresh frozen plasma in a 1:1 ratio), if needed, to maintain a central pulse.
- Consider pelvic splint (e.g. SAM splint).
- Draw out any deformed limbs to length (e.g. with Kendrick splint).
- Control any obvious external haemorrhage.

- Package patient skin to scoop, wrap/keep warm, and air lift to nearest major trauma centre.
- Ventilate to normocapnia. Hyperventilating will lead to hypocapnia and therefore intracerebral vasoconstriction which will reduce cerebral perfusion.
- Keep head up at about 30 degrees.
- Manage the presumed coumarin or novel oral anticoagulant-induced coagulopathy: Octaplex®/ Beriplex® (prothrombin complex concentrate)—idarucizumab if presumed to be on dabigatran (in-hospital).
- Fresh frozen plasma (with a blood in a 1:1 ratio if needed).
- Vitamin K 5–10 mg intravenous, if available.
- Give tranexamic acid 1 G intravenous.
- Assuming raised intracranial pressure, consider 500 ml of 20% mannitol or 150 ml boluses of 3% hypertonic saline.

A3.

The lethal triad of death, in the context of a trauma patient, is the concurrence of hypothermia, coagulopathy, and metabolic acidosis.

Bleeding results in impaired delivery of oxygen to the tissues. This contributes to metabolic acidosis consistent with decrease in oxidative metabolism. Exsanguination and prolonged exposure to the environment, results in hypothermia. Hypothermia disrupts the coagulation cascade which results in further bleeding and worsening of the metabolic acidosis.

It is a self-perpetuating cycle that carries a higher mortality. The primary aims are therefore to resuscitate the patient (restore oxygen delivery to the tissues and cells at the mitochondrial level), to keep the patient warm and reverse coagulopathy (PCC, TXA, FFP, platelets, cryoprecipitate (cryostat-2), vitamin K).

Further Reading

Mercer SJ, Kingston EV, Jones CPL. The trauma call. *BMJ*. 2018;361 k2272.
Rossaint R, Bouillon B, Cerny V, Coats TJ, Duranteau J, Fernández-Mondéjar E, et al. The European guideline on management of major bleeding and coagulopathy following trauma: fourth edition. *Critical Care*. 2016;20:100.

SAQ 4 **Head Injury**

A 22-year-old male is brought in after an assault. He localizes to pain, makes incomprehensible noises, and does not open his eyes. He has a large wound to his right occipital scalp and bruising over the right mastoid. He has no other obvious injuries. He smells strongly of alcohol and has vomit on his clothing.

His pulse is 60 beats per minute, and his BP is 90/60 mm Hg. His oxygen saturation on room air is 95%.

Q1. What is his Glasgow Coma Score?

Q2. What indications does this patient have for an immediate computed tomography (CT) scan of his brain, according to the National Institute for Health and Care Excellence (NICE) guidelines?

Q3. Within a few minutes the patient's blood pressure increases to 200/120 mm Hg. He becomes bradycardic. His right pupil is now fixed and dilated. Explain the pathophysiology of what is occurring, with reference to any relevant neuroanatomy?

Answers

A1.

His Glasgow Coma Score = 8 (Eyes 1, Voice 2, Motor 5).

A2.

Indications for CT head scan in this case are:

- Signs of base of skull fracture
- GCS <13 at presentation

According to NICE guidelines, the following features mandate immediate CT head in adults:

- GCS <13 on initial assessment in the ED
- GCS <15 two hours after the injury
- Open or depressed skull fracture
- Signs of base of skull fracture (haemotympanum, 'panda' eyes, CSF otorrhoea, CSF rhinorrhoea, Battle's sign of ecchymosis overlying the mastoid process)
- Post-traumatic seizure
- Focal neurological deficit
- More than one episode of vomiting
- More than 30 minutes of retrograde amnesia
- Loss of consciousness only if one or more of the following present:
  - Age >65 years
  - Coagulopathy (history of bleeding, clotting disorder, concurrent anticoagulation therapy)
  - Dangerous mechanism of injury (e.g. pedestrian vs. a vehicle, fall from height more than one metre, ejected from vehicle)

A3.

Raised intracranial pressure causes the uncus, the innermost part, of the temporal lobe to herniate downwards compressing the ipsilateral oculomotor nerve.

Cushing's response results from compression of the midbrain as it herniates through the foramen magnum. It is initiated by the hypothalamus. The hypothalamus activates the sympathetic nervous system, causing peripheral vasoconstriction and an increase in cardiac output. These two effects serve to increase arterial blood pressure. When arterial blood pressure exceeds the intracranial pressure, blood flow to the brain is restored. However, the increased arterial blood pressure stimulates the baroreceptors in the carotid bodies, thus inducing a bradycardia.

Further Reading

NICE. *Head Injury: Assessment and Early Management CG176.* 2017. Available from: https://www.nice.org.uk/guidance/cg176

SAQ 5 Subdural Haematoma

A 58-year-old man is found unresponsive in the park. You note a haematoma over his right forehead and decide to perform a CT head which is shown in Fig. 20.3.

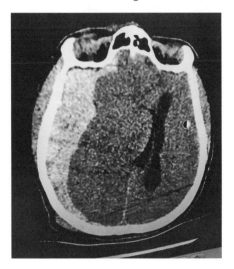

Fig. 20.3

Q1. What is the diagnosis?

Q2. Your Foundation Year 2 doctor (FY2) mentions that this patient is on warfarin. What drug can you give to rapidly reverse warfarin?

Q3. What can be given to reduce the intracranial pressure?

Answers

A1.

The CT scan shows acute subdural haemorrhage with mid-line shift (owing to increased pressure on the side of the injury notice how the falx cerebri is pushed across to the opposite side). Subdural haemorrhage is more common than extradural haemorrhage. It results from shearing forces that tear the bridging veins between the dural and arachnoid meningeal layers. They tend to have a concave appearance on their innermost surface (as opposed to extradural haemorrhage, which has a classic convex inner surface). Subdural bleeds also tend to be more diffuse and cover a larger portion of the cerebral hemispheres than extradural bleeds, as they cross suture lines. Risk factors for subdural haemorrhage are older age, alcoholism, and use of anticoagulant medication. There is brain atrophy in elderly patients which enlarges the subdural space and places more tension on the bridging veins making them more vulnerable to injury.

Furthermore, injuries not involving the brain parenchyma are described an 'extra-axial' (e.g. sub-dural, extradural, and subarachnoid haemorrhage) and those directly involving the brain parenchyma are 'intra-axial' (i.e. intracerebral haemorrhage).

A2.

Prothrombin complex concentrate (contains factors II, VII, IX, and X). The dose is 50 units/kg intravenous.

A3.

Give 0.25–2 g/kg of mannitol over 20–60 minutes. Mannitol is available in 10% or 20% strength. An easily remembered dose for a 70 kg patient is 200 ml of 20% mannitol (equivalent to 0.57 g/kg). An alternative is hypertonic saline (150 ml aliquots of 3%).

Both mannitol and hypertonic saline reduce intracranial pressure. They do this by producing an intravascular hyperosmolality. Hypertonic saline achieves this simply by the direct introduction of hypertonic solution to the circulation and mannitol by inducing an osmotic diuresis. In terms of clinical benefit, the evidence is not particularly strong in favour of one over the other, but currently the evidence leans slightly in favour of hypertonic saline.

Further Reading

Grande AW. Subdural haematoma. *BMJ Best Practice*. 2018. Available from: https://bestpractice.bmj.com/topics/en-gb/416

SAQ 6 **Open Tibia Fracture**

A 48-year-old motorcyclist is brought in to the resuscitation room of a major trauma centre. You have completed a primary survey and he is haemodynamically normal but noted to have an open tibia fracture.

Q1. List four things you would do prior to definitive management.
Q2. List three signs of arterial injury within the limb.
Q3. List three forms of pain control (include route and dose where applicable).

Answers

A1.

Initial management includes

- Analgesia, which may involve titrated opiate administration
- Tetanus prophylaxis
- Intravenous antibiotics (with reference to local guidelines)
- Splint if necessary
- Assess neurovascular status distally

A2.

The signs of arterial injury within the limb include:

- Pallor
- Pulselessness
- Perishingly cold
- Power loss (paresis or paralysis)
- Paraesthesiae
- Pain

A3.

Relevant methods of pain control include:

- Intravenous morphine (5 mg increments titrated to effect, with antiemetic)
- Intravenous ketamine (1 mg/kg)
- Entonox® (50:50 nitrous oxide: oxygen mixture)

Further Reading

Mundi R, Chaudhry H, Niroopam G, Petrisor B, Bhandari M. Open tibial fractures: updated guidelines for management. *Bone & Joint Research*. 2014;3:161–3.

SAQ 7 **Epicondylitis**

The next minors card says 'elbow problem for 3–4 weeks'.

Q1. What are the clinical findings characteristic of tennis elbow?
Q2. What are the clinical findings characteristic of golfer's elbow?
Q3. What is the advice would you give in the emergency department?

Answers

A1.

Tenderness is expected approximately 1 cm distal and anterior to the lateral epicondyle. Resisted wrist/digit extension causes pain as does passive wrist flexion with an extended elbow (the medical terms for tennis elbow is lateral epicondylitis).

A2.

Tenderness is expected 5 mm distal and anterior to the medial epicondyle along the medial elbow. Resisted forearm pronation and wrist flexion causes pain (the medical terms for golfer's elbow is medial epicondylitis).

A3.

Advice at discharge include six weeks of rest, ice, and modified activity. For the first few weeks non-steroidal anti-inflammatory drugs (NSAIDs) can be used to good effect. Forearm strapping in lateral epicondylitis can be helpful. If no improvement in 6 weeks, a physiotherapist can be recommended. If no improvements are found, corticosteroid injections are often adopted although the evidence base for this is variable. Other non-surgical approaches exist but at 6–12 months a surgical option may be considered appropriate.

Further Reading

Ahmad Z, Siddiqui N, Malik SS, Abdus-Samee M, Tytherleigh-Strong G, Rushton N. Lateral epicondylitis. A review of pathology and management. *The Bone & Joint Journal*. 2013;95B:1158–64.

SAQ 8 **Major Head Injury**

A 23-year-old motorcyclist has been brought to the resuscitation room with a major head injury.

Q1. List five potential causes of secondary brain injury.
Q2. List four methods that can be instituted to reduce the impact of secondary brain injury.
Q3. Define what is meant by impact brain apnoea.

Answers

A1.

Secondary brain injury may be related to:

- Hypoxaemia
- Hypotension
- Seizure
- Cerebral oedema
- Intracranial haematoma

A2.

The impact of secondary brain injury can be minimized by the following interventions:

- Secure the airway
- Ventilatory support
- Volume replacement
- Control of raised intracranial pressure (mannitol or hypertonic saline)

A3.

Impact brain apnoea is a phenomenon that most likely results in significant morbidity and mortality following a head injury. On impact, there is an episode of apnoea, which can exacerbate secondary brain injury. On recovery, there is a period of very abnormal ventilation. It requires early intervention with rapid sequence induction and ventilatory support.

Further Reading

NICE. *Head Injury: Assessment and Early Management CG176.* 2014. Available from: https://www.nice.org.uk/guidance/cg176

SAQ 9 **Head Injury**

An 80-year-old lady, with a history of falls, tripped while descending the staircase at home. She stumbled on the final step and fell, hitting her head against the wall. She is on Rivaroxaban for atrial fibrillation but has no other past medical history. Her neighbour, unable to make contact with her, called the ambulance. She was brought into your emergency department, a trauma unit, on a scoop with her neck immobilized. Her GCS is 14. Vital signs are as follows: blood pressure 144/85 mm Hg, pulse rate 91 beats per minute, arterial oxygen saturation 94% air, and capillary blood glucose 5.9 mmol/L. Apart from a laceration to the left side of her head there appear to be no other injuries

Q1. Outline your approach to the initial management of this patient including any imaging you require. List four key interventions.

Q2. Her CT brain is shown in Fig. 20.4. Describe the abnormality.

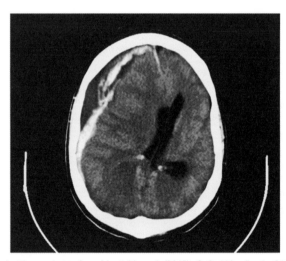

Fig. 20.4 Reproduced with permission from Manji, H. et al. (2015). *Oxford Handbook of Neurology*. 2nd ed. Oxford University Press. © Oxford University Press 2014. Reproduced with permission of the licensor via PLSClear.

Q3. The patient drops her Glasgow Coma Score to 9. The blood pressure is now 170/100 mm Hg, and the pulse rate is 60/minute. Describe how you will manage her.

Answers

A1.

Team approach following the ABCDE principles (Airway, Breathing, Circulation, Disability, Exposure):

- Listen carefully to ambulance handover.
- Get patient off scoop onto emergency department trolley and commence primary survey:

- ◆ Assess airway. Provide O_2. Ensure anaesthetic support is available. May need adjuncts. Need to consider prepping for rapid sequence induction in this clinical context.
- ◆ Maintain immobilization of the cervical spine.
- ◆ Pulse oximetry probe, blood pressure cuff, and cardiac monitoring in place.
- ◆ Establish intravenous access (or intraosseous if difficult). Take bloods including glucose, venous blood gases, blood counts, urea and electrolytes.
- ◆ Intravenous crystalloid not indicated and potentially harmful in the bleeding trauma patient. Product of choice in exsanguinating trauma is blood (with fresh frozen plasma in a 1:1 ratio), titrated to a central pulse ('permissive hypotension').
- ◆ eFAST scan (to look for possible intraperitoneal and pericardial blood and to exclude a pneumothorax).
- ◆ Plain films of chest and pelvis to screen for any obvious life-threatening injuries that may require immediate intervention. There may even be pathology on chest X-ray to explain fall (i.e. pneumonia).
- ◆ Arrange a minimum of a CT head and neck. CT head to pelvis would be preferred.
- Give analgesia if required (intravenous paracetamol and/or small incremental aliquots of morphine with concomitant antiemetic therapy).
- Keep patient warm throughout.
- Log-roll only if stable to do so. Rarely adds anything particularly if patient going for CT.

A2.

The CT scan shows an acute on chronic left sided subdural haematoma with ventricular effacement and mid-line shift (extra-axial bleed). Notice how the falx cerebri is shifted over to the opposite side of the injury ('mass effect'). Notice the diffuse low attenuation (darker) area beneath the skull on the left side (right on the picture as you see it). This represents a chronic subdural haematoma. The superimposed higher attenuation area (brighter) represents acute blood.

A3.

The interventions required include:

- Rapid sequence induction. Virtually simultaneous administration of a hypnotic agent with a neuromuscular blocking agent (e.g. propofol + rocuronium or ketamine + rocuronium). Consider an adjuvant dose of fentanyl. Propofol is neuroprotective and ketamine not shown to exacerbate the raised intracranial pressure.
- Ventilate patient to normocapnia. Hyperventilating the patient will drive hypocapnia and intracerebral vasoconstriction worsening cerebral ischaemia. Hypoventilating, the patient will drive hypercapnia precipitating intracerebral vasodilatation and raise the increased intracranial pressure (ICP) further.
- Patient managed and nursed in a 30-degree head up position.
- Consider a dose of tranexamic acid 1 g intravenous. (The CRASH 3 trial is ongoing). Discuss other options with the on-call haematology Consultant. If on warfarin, then would require Octaplex® STAT.
- Consider a dose of either mannitol or hypertonic saline (there is no standard or NICE guideline). Both agents increase intravascular osmolarity (mannitol by inducing a diuresis and hypertonic by adding solute to the circulation). Doses: mannitol—500 ml of 20% (100 g) infused rapidly; hypertonic— 150 ml boluses of 3%. No strong evidence but favour seems to lean slightly towards hypertonic.
- Transfer patient to a major trauma centre via critical transfer ambulance and with airway trained escort.

Further Reading

NICE. *Head Injury: Assessment and Early Management CG176*. 2014. Available from: https://www.nice.org.uk/guidance/cg176

SAQ 10 **Smoke Inhalation**

A 60-year-old female has been extricated from a smoke-filled room following a house fire.

Q1. List four signs of major inhalational airway injury.
Q2. What is the immediate management (list three interventions)?
Q3. What are the indications for tracheal intubation?

Answers

A1.

Major inhalational injury to the airways can be indicated by:

- Hoarse voice
- Facial burns
- Singed facial or nasal hair
- Soot staining of nasal or oral mucosa
- Carbonaceous sputum
- Stridor

A2.

The immediate management of inhalational airway injury includes:

- High-flow oxygen via non-rebreathing mask
- Consideration of early intubation
- Ventilatory support

A3.

Tracheal intubation is indicated in the presence of:

- Impending or actual upper airway obstruction
- Reduced level of consciousness
- Increasing hypoxaemia

Further Reading

Walker PF, Buehner MF, Wood LA, Boyer NL, Driscoll IR, Lundy JB, et al. Diagnosis and management of inhalation injury: an updated review *Critical Care*. 2015;19:351.

Chapter 21 **Urology**

SAQ 1 **Acute Urinary Retention**

A 66-year-old man is sent to the emergency department directly from his general practitioner's surgery. He is unable to pass urine and is in considerable pain. You ask one of your junior colleagues to prepare a tray for catheterization while you clerk the gentleman. A focused history reveals the cause is very likely urinary outflow obstruction from benign prostatic hypertrophy.

Q1. List four further causes of acute urinary retention.
Q2. The patient is anxious to know what the next step is. What advice will you give?
Q3. What is the mechanism of action of tamsulosin, and what is the recommended dose?

Answers

A1.

Causes of acute urinary retention include:

- Outflow obstruction caused by cancer of the prostate or prostatitis
- Urethral blockage by stones or blood clots
- Urethral stricture
- Constipation
- Tumour within the pelvis
- Perineal pain caused by, for example, herpetic infection or postoperative pain
- Medication: anticholinergics, tricyclic antidepressants, antihistamines, antipsychotic medications, atropine, disopyramide, ipratropium, ephedrine and pseudoephedrine, opioid analgesia, anaesthetic agents

Urinary retention can be obstructive, inflammatory, neurological, or pharmacological (due to anticholinergic or alpha-adrenergic agonist agents). Obstructive causes are at or distal to the bladder neck.

A2.

Urine needs to be tested for the presence of blood and for any evidence of infection, which can precipitate acute urinary retention.

Early urethral catheterization, with documentation of residual volume is useful in quantifying the degree of bladder outlet obstruction.

If the urethra is impassable, suprapubic cystostomy is indicated.

Patients can usually be discharged home with an indwelling urethral catheter (provided they are haemodynamically stable and that there is no frank haematuria), attached to a leg bag, and followed up in the outpatient urology clinic for trial without catheter, usually led by nurse specialists. The patient will also need to be commenced on oral tamsulosin.

A3.

Tamsulosin is an alpha-adrenergic blocker (α_1–blocker). The dose is 0.4 mg (400 micrograms). It relaxes smooth muscle; it is also indicated in benign prostatic hyperplasia and to facilitate the passage of small ureteral stones. It must be used for at least 24 hours before the catheter is removed. Once removed, several hours are required to confirm that voiding is normal.

Further Reading

Fitzpatrick JM, Kirby RS. Management of acute urinary retention. *BJU International*. 2006;97 Suppl 2:16–20.

SAQ 2 **Urine Dipstick**

A 33-year-old non-pregnant lady presents with one week of dysuria. She says she could not get an appointment with her general practitioner. The triage nurse has done a urine dipstick which showed 'leucocytes +'.

Q1. Did this lady need a urine dipstick?
Q2. Considering the urine dipstick alone, how would the results 'leucocytes +' and/or 'nitrites +' affect the likelihood of bacteriuria?
Q3. What would your choice and duration of antibiotics be?

Answers

A1.

Yes. This lady has less than three symptoms of a urinary tract infection and is under the age of 65 years. She could be treated empirically if she had three or more symptoms.

A2.

With one clinical symptom present, the detection of both leucocytes and nitrites in the urine has a positive predictive value for bacteriuria of about 80%. The presence of leucocytes alone carries a low positive predictive value (about 30%). The presence of nitrites alone carries about a 60% positive predictive value. Although a negative test does not rule out bacteriuria, it takes the probability down to 20%.

A3.

Follow local guidelines, but either trimethoprim, 200 mg twice daily orally, or nitrofurantoin, 50 mg four times daily for 3 days.

Further Reading

NICE. *Urinary Tract Infections in Adults QS90*. 2015. Available from: https://www.nice.org.uk/guidance/qs90
SIGN. *Management of Suspected Bacterial Urinary Tract Infections in Adults*. 2012. Available from: https://www.sign.ac.uk/sign-88-management-of-suspected-bacterial-urinary-tract-infection-in-adults.html

SAQ 3 **Acute Kidney Injury**

You have admitted an 85-year-old female to the clinical decision unit with a history of recent diarrhoea and vomiting. Blood tests confirm acute kidney injury.

Q1. List two diagnostic criteria for acute kidney injury.

Q2. What three management measures might be indicated for your patient?

Q3. List three types of renal replacement therapy.

Answers

A1.

Diagnostic criteria for acute kidney injury are:

- Increase in serum creatinine >26.5 µmol/L (0.3 mg/dl) within 48 hours
- Increase in serum creatinine to at least 1.5 times baseline (known or presumed to have occurred within previous seven days)
- Urine output <0.5 ml/kg/hour for at least six hours

A2.

Management of acute kidney injury involves:

- Rapid correction of hypovolaemia and restoration of haemodynamic status with intravenous crystalloid
- Prompt treatment of sepsis
- Avoidance of nephrotoxins
- Adjustment of the dose of renal excreted drugs (digoxin, low molecular weight heparins, opioids, penicillins)
- Correction of hyperkalaemia (must act promptly in the presence of electrocardiogram (ECG) changes)

A3.

Types of renal replacement therapy include:

- Intermittent haemodialysis
- Continuous renal replacement therapy: veno-venous haemofiltration
- Peritoneal dialysis
- Renal transplantation

Further Reading

NICE. *Acute Kidney Injury: Prevention, Detection and Management CG169*. 2013. Available from: https://www.nice.org.uk/guidance/cg169

SAQ 4 **Priapism**

A 28-year-old male presents very concerned about a persistent and painful penile erection he has now had overnight for seven hours. You suspect priapism.

Q1. Define priapism.
Q2. Describe three treatment options.
Q3. How is priapism characterized?

Answers

A1.

Priapism refers to an involuntary penile erection that has been persistent for more than six hours and is unrelated to sexual stimulation.

A2.

Treatment options for priapism include:

- Local ice
- Gentle walking
- Analgesia
- Aspiration of blood from the corpus cavernosa under local anaesthesia, using a 50 ml syringe and a fine needle (e.g. a 22-gauge butterfly type needle). The corpora can be washed out with saline at the same time
- Intracavernosal phenylephrine (alpha-adrenergic agonist) injection
- Oral terbutaline
- Treatment of the underlying cause (e.g. sickle cell disease)

A3.

Priapism can be of either a low-flow (ischaemic) or a high-flow (non-ischaemic) type:

- Low-flow priapism is the most common, resulting from failure of venous outflow. Associated causes are sickle cell disease, cervical spine trauma, drugs (e.g. calcium channel blockers, cocaine, anti-impotence treatment, anticoagulants)
- High-flow priapism results from uncontrolled arterial inflow. Most commonly from local trauma

Further reading

Dubin J, Davis JE. Penile emergencies. *Emergency Medicine Clinics of North America.* 2011;29:485–99.

SAQ 5 **Acute Scrotal Pain**

A 15-year-old boy attends the paediatric emergency department with an acutely painful scrotum, for the last four hours. He reports pain on and off for several days but was too embarrassed to tell anyone.

Q1. What are the likely differential diagnoses? What features in the history and examination would help differentiate each diagnosis?

Q2. List four non-bacterial causative agents in epididymo-orchitis.

Q3. Outline the management of acute bacterial epididymo-orchitis.

Answers

A1.

Box 21.1 outlines the differential diagnosis.

Diagnosis	Features
Torsion of the testes	Acute onset <12 hours, common in children and 12–18-year-olds, rare >30 years, in 25% of cases no sudden onset of symptoms, intermittent torsion can occur. Examination reveals a tender swollen testis which lies on a different axis to the normal side. The affected testis may be higher and it may not be possible to 'get above it'.
Epididymo- orchitis	Patients tend to be older, the spermatic cord is tender and swollen, there is often urethritis, often sexually active, and associated with STIs.

A2.

Non-bacterial causes of epididymo-orchitis include:

- Chlamydia trachomatis
- Mumps
- Drugs—amiodarone
- Fungal—cryptococcal
- Parasitic—filariasis

Bacterial causes include:

- *Neisseria gonorrhoeae*
- *Escherichia coli*
- Pseudomonas
- Coliforms
- Klebsiella
- Tuberculosis

A3.

Urethral swabs for microscopy and culture—looking for diplococci.

Bed rest

Scrotal supports

Analgesia

Antibiotics—to cover for sexually transmitted infections if heterosexual male, cover coliforms if homosexual, and if secondary to urinary tract infection ciprofloxacin

For patients aged 35 years or younger, most often the causative organism is a sexually transmitted pathogen (*Chlamydia trachomatis; Neisseria gonorrhoeae*); while above the age of 35 years, non-sexually transmitted Gram-negative enteric pathogens causing urinary tract infections predominate

Further Reading

Srinath H. Acute scrotal pain. *Australian Family Physician*. 2013;42:790–2.

SAQ 6 **Hydronephrosis**

A 55-year-old male presents to the emergency department with acute left loin pain. It has been present on and off for several months but is worse today. His is renal ultrasound is shown in Fig. 21.1.

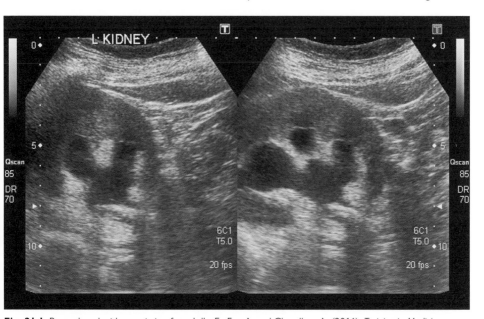

Fig. 21.1 Reproduced with permission from Jolly, E., Fry, A. and Chaudhry, A. (2016). *Training in Medicine*. Oxford University Press. © Oxford University Press 2016. Reproduced with permission of the licensor via PLSClear.

Q1. What is the abnormality on the scan?
Q2. List three possible causes of this appearance.
Q3. What surgical procedure should be considered and what is the indication?

Answers

A1.

The ultrasound shows gross hydronephrosis of the left kidney.

A2.

Possible causes of hydronephrosis are:

- Calculus disease
- Neoplastic disease
- Previous trauma

- Previous surgery
- Previous radiotherapy
- Retroperitoneal fibrosis

A3.

Percutaneous nephrostomy is required for temporary urinary diversion associated with urinary obstruction, prior to definitive treatment.

Further Reading

Türk C, Knoll T, Petrik A, Sarika K, Skolarikos A, Straub M, Seitz C. *Guidelines on Urolithiasis*. European Association of Urology, 2015. Available from: https://uroweb.org/wp-content/uploads/EAU-Guidelines-Urolithiasis-2015-v2.pdf

SAQ 7 **Ureteric Stone**

You have requested a CT-KUB scan for a 32-year-old male presenting with sharp intermittent right-sided loin pain associated with microscopic haematuria. A 5 mm stone is seen in the right distal ureter.

Q1. What are the options for medical expulsive therapy for this patient?
Q2. Under what circumstances would admission to hospital be required?
Q3. What are the treatment options for emergency decompression of an infected obstructed urinary tract?

Answers

A1.

The options for medical expulsive therapy are:

- Alpha 1 adrenergic blockers: tamsulosin 400 mcg daily for ten days
- Calcium channel blockers: nifedipine XL 30 mg daily

A2.

Admission to hospital is required with:

- Coexisting sepsis
- Obstructed urinary tract (presence of a hydronephrosis)
- Uncontrolled pain
- High-grade obstruction of a solitary or transplanted kidney
- Impaired renal function, with acute kidney injury

A3.

Percutaneous nephrostomy or retrograde insertion of a ureteral JJ stent are required for emergency decompression of an infected obstructed urinary tract.

SAQ 8 **Haematuria**

An 80-year-old male presents with frank haematuria. He is passing clots via the urethra, and on examination is noted to be in acute urinary retention. He is on warfarin for atrial fibrillation.

Q1. What is your initial management?

Q2. How would you manage his therapeutic anticoagulation?

Q3. The patient is admitted to the surgical assessment unit (SAU). What surgical procedure is indicated for assessment and treatment?

Answers

A1.

A three-way catheter should be inserted into the bladder. The catheter has three ports: one to inflate the catheter balloon; one to allow free drainage of urine from the bladder; and one to allow rapid infusion of fluids into the bladder

A2.

Follow local guidelines for management of anticoagulation, but generally speaking:

- If patient becomes unstable then warfarin requires rapid reversal with Octaplex® 50 units/kg
- Otherwise measure the INR:
  + If INR >8: even if asymptomatic warfarin must be withheld for 1–2 doses and reintroduced when INR <4. Vitamin K 5 mg intravenous must be given in the interim for partial reversal.
  + If INR 4–8 and bleeding then the aforementioned advice applies.
  + If INR 4–8 and *not* actively bleeding then warfarin may be withheld for 1–2 doses and reintroduced when INR< 4 but vitamin K is not required.

A3.

Surgical options include:

- Flexible cystoscopy
- Rigid cystoscopy under general anaesthesia and biopsy-if abnormality on flexible cystoscopy

SAQ 9 **Acute Scrotal Pain 2**

A 22-year-old male attends the emergency department with the acute onset of pain and swelling in the right scrotum. You consider the possibility of testicular torsion.

Q1. What features on clinical examination will support the diagnosis?
Q2. List three conditions in the differential diagnosis.
Q3. What is the definitive management for testicular torsion?

Answers

A1.

Testicular torsion is suggested by the presence of:

• Scrotal enlargement and tenderness, as opposed to epididymal tenderness
• Transverse lie of the affected testis
• Loss of cremasteric reflex on the affected side

A2.

The differential diagnosis of an acute scrotum includes the following:

• Acute epididymo-orchitis
• Torsion of appendix testis
• Testicular tumour with haemorrhage
• Trauma with scrotal haematocele

A3.

The definitive management is urgent scrotal exploration within 4–6 hours of onset of pain and bilateral testicular fixation.

Further Reading

Somani BK, Watson G, Townell N. Testicular torsion. *BMJ.* 2010;341:c3213.

Chapter 22 **Vascular Emergencies**

SAQ 1 **Massive and Submassive Pulmonary Embolism**

You are called to the resuscitation room as a 37-year-old female has been brought in as a priority call. The history is of sudden collapse and hypotension, on the background of recently diagnosed deep vein thrombosis. You initiate resuscitation measures, and suspect that this presentation is caused by a massive pulmonary embolus.

Q1. How quickly should CTPA (CT-pulmonary angiogram) ideally be performed in massive pulmonary embolism (PE)?

Q2. Is there a survival benefit of thrombolysis for those with submassive PE demonstrating right ventricular dysfunction?

Q3. What percentage of patients admitted with non-traumatic electromechanical dissociation or asystole turn out to have a massive PE?

Answers

A1.

CTPA should be performed within one hour of presentation.

A2.

There is no demonstrable survival benefit and the literature still points toward thrombolysis being reserved only for massive PE with circulatory collapse.

A3.

50%.

NICE guidelines outline the current approach to thrombolysis in pulmonary embolus as well as management of non-massive PE.

Further Reading

Konstantinides SV, Torbicki A, Agnelli G, Danchin N, Fitzmaurice D, Galiè N, et al. 2014 ESC guidelines on the diagnosis and management of acute pulmonary embolism. *European Heart Journal*. 2014;35:3033–80.

NICE. *Venous Thromboembolic Diseases: Diagnosis, Management, and Thrombophilia Testing CG144*. 2012. Available from: https://www.nice.org.uk/guidance/cg144

SAQ 2 **Aortic Dissection**

A 25-year-old male attends with severe acute central chest pain which caused him to collapse. He is pale and clammy, tachycardic, and hypertensive.

Q1. What is the most important likely diagnosis?
Q2. Describe one commonly used classification system.
Q3. How does treatment vary according to the classification used? What drugs are used in the medical management?

Answers

A1.

Acute aortic dissection. This should be considered in the presence of acute onset of severe pain, which may be located in the anterior chest (retrosternal), interscapular region, or lower back. The pain is typically stabbing, tearing, or ripping, and maximal at the onset. Pain may migrate along the path of progression of the dissection. Dissection may cause end-organ ischaemia, leading to myocardial infarction, stroke, paraplegia, ischaemic bowel, acute kidney injury, or acute limb ischaemia.

A2.

There are two major classifications, although the Stanford classification is used more frequently.

De Bakey: The dissection may involve both ascending & descending aorta along with the intervening aortic arch (I), ascending aorta alone (II), or descending aorta alone (III)
Stanford:

Stanford A—involves ascending aorta alone or both ascending and descending aorta (De Bakey I or II)
Stanford B—involves only descending aorta (De Bakey III)

A3.

Stanford A—requires surgical management, which involves graft replacement of the involved thoracic aorta. In addition, aortic valve replacement and coronary artery reimplantation may occasionally be required.
    Stanford B—medical management is initially indicated. Intravenous beta-blockers are used to lower blood pressure and pressure load, thereby minimizing the risk of extension or rupture of the dissection. Intravenous beta-blockade should aim for a target heart rate less than 60/minute and a target blood pressure less than 120/80 mm Hg. It is important to maintain an adequate urine output. Esmolol 0.5 mg/kg loading dose over 2–5 minutes, followed by 0.10–0.20 mg/kg/minute infusion is

usually indicated. If the blood pressure remains high despite adequate beta-blockade, a vasodilator, such as sodium nitroprusside or glyceryl trinitrate, can be infused intravenously. Surgical management is indicated if the dissection propagates in the presence of optimal medical management.

Further Reading

Erbel R, Aboyans V, Boileau C, Bossone E, Bartolomeo RD, Eggebrecht H. 2014 ESC guidelines on the diagnosis and treatment of aortic diseases. *European Heart Journal*. 2014;35:2873–926.

SAQ 3 Acute Lower Limb Ischaemia

A 62-year-old female attends with an acutely painful left foot and calf. She has no history of trauma. She describes a constant severe dull ache and has required 10 mg of morphine from the ambulance with only slight relief.

Q1. What is the most likely diagnosis?
Q2. What simple investigation can confirm the diagnosis?
Q3. Outline the management of this patient (list three options).

Answers

A1.

Acute ischaemia of the left leg is most likely. The six Ps of acute arterial ischaemia include:

- Pain
- Pallor
- Pulselessness
- Paraesthesia
- Poikilothermia (or perishing with cold)
- Paralysis

The clinical features are more severe and progress more rapidly with embolic (cardiac or arterial in origin) occlusions. In thrombotic occlusions superimposed on chronic peripheral arterial disease, the presence of collaterals reduces the severity of presentation.

A2.

Bedside hand-held Doppler examination may show the absence of audible arterial signals.

The diagnosis is usually confirmed with contrast-enhanced CT arteriography, or magnetic resonance arteriography. Digital subtraction arteriography has been regarded as the diagnostic gold standard, but is an invasive procedure involving direct injection of contrast into the artery.

A3.

Management includes:

- Analgesia, often opiates
- Heparinisation
- Urgent vascular referral for evaluation and treatment, which may include mechanical (e.g. aspiration thrombectomy, balloon catheter embolectomy) or pharmacological recanalization (e.g. thrombolysis), or surgical therapy (e.g. thromboembolectomy, vascular bypass surgery)

Further Reading

Aboyans V, Ricco J-B, Bartelink MEL, Björck M, Brodmann M, Cohnert T, et al. 2017 ESC Guidelines on the diagnosis and treatment of peripheral arterial diseases. *European Heart Journal*. 2018;39:763–816.

SAQ 4 **Ruptured Abdominal Aortic Aneurysm**

A 75-year-old male with a leaking abdominal aortic aneurysm requires transfer to a tertiary vascular centre.

Q1. List three initial management priorities.
Q2. What is the recommended time limit for transfer?
Q3. What are the definitive treatment options?

Answers

A1.

The initial management includes:

- Large-bore intravenous access in both upper limbs
- Permissive hypotension, maintaining a systolic blood pressure ≥70 mm Hg
- Bedside ultrasound to confirm presence of an abdominal aortic aneurysm
- If an alternative diagnosis is likely, CT scan prior to transfer with electronic image transmission
- Rapid coordinated time-critical transfer

A2.

The time limit for transfer is within 30 minutes of diagnosis.

A3.

Definitive treatment options for leaking aortic aneurysms include either:

- Open repair
- EVAR (endovascular aneurysm repair)

Further Reading

Chaikof EL, Dalman RL, Eskandari MK, Jackson BM, Lee WA, Mansour MA, et al. The Society for Vascular Surgery practice guidelines on the care of patients with an abdominal aortic aneurysm. *Journal of Vascular Surgery.* 2018;67:2–77.

SAQ 5 Abdominal Aortic Aneurysm

Q1. Your Foundation Year 2 (FY2) trainee is keen to learn about using the ultrasound machine in the emergency department and shows you the abdominal scan shown in Fig. 22.1a: label the three identified areas.

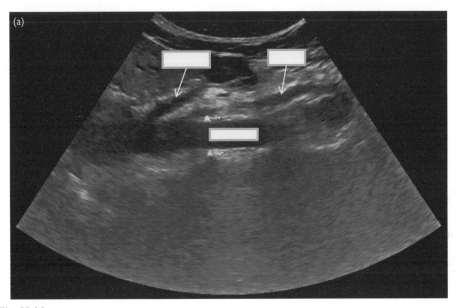

Fig. 22.1A

Q2. Where are most abdominal aortic aneurysms found?

Q3. What measurement is used to diagnose an aortic aneurysm?

Answers

A1.

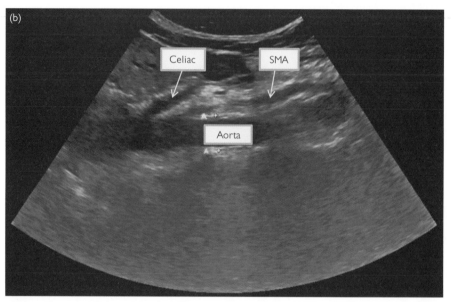

Fig. 221B

A2.

The majority (90–95%) of AAA are situated below the renal arteries. In order to exclude an AAA on ultrasound, you need to visualize the aorta from the above the coeliac axis to beyond the bifurcation into iliac vessels.

A3.

An aorta with an anteroposterior diameter of more than 3 cm is defined as an aneurysm.

Further Reading

RCEM. *Core (Level 1) Ultrasound Curriculum*. Available from: https://www.rcem.ac.uk/docs/Training/1.14.5%20 RCEM-EMUS-booklet%20(3).pdf

SAQ 6 **Pulmonary Embolism 2**

A 52-year-old man presents with pleuritic chest pain and no other symptoms. He has no relevant past medical or surgical history, takes no medications, and has been well in himself leading up to this presentation. His observations are as follows: heart rate 80/minute; blood pressure 131/82 mm Hg; oxygen saturation 96%; respiratory rate 12/minute.

Q1. Can pulmonary embolism be ruled out in this gentleman using the Pulmonary Embolism Rule-Out Criteria (PERC) rule?

Q2. What other key feature of the assessment is required for the PERC rule to be used accurately?

Q3. What features are used in the Wells score for pulmonary embolism which are not specifically found when calculating using the PERC rule?

Answers

A1.

No. He is over 50 years old. The PERC rule can only be used to rule out pulmonary embolus if the score is 0 as this takes the chance down to less than 2%. The parameters which must be met for a score of zero are:

- Age less than 50
- Heart rate less than 100
- Oxygen saturations more than 95%
- No previous venous thromboembolism
- No trauma or surgery in the preceding 4 weeks
- No haemoptysis
- No exogenous oestrogen
- No unilateral leg swelling

Reproduced from Kline, J.A. et al. Clinical criteria to prevent unnecessary diagnostic testing in emergency department patients with suspected pulmonary embolism. *Journal of Thrombosis and Haemostasis*, 2004, 2: 1247-1255. https://doi.org/10.1111/j.1538-7836.2004.00790.x. Copyright © 2004, John Wiley and Sons.

A2.

The physician assessing the patient must have used clinical judgement (gestalt) to indicate that the patient is at low risk of pulmonary embolus before using the score.

A3.

Specific features of the Wells score include:

- Pulmonary embolism is most or equally likely diagnosis
- Malignancy (with treatment within 6 months) or palliative
- Immobilization for at least 3 days

The full score is:

- clinical signs and symptoms of deep vein thrombosis—3 points
- pulmonary embolism is most likely or equally likely diagnosis—3 points
- heart rate >100—1.5 points
- immobilization at least 3 days, or surgery in the previous 4 weeks—1.5 points
- previous, objectively diagnosed PE or DVT—1.5 points
- haemoptysis—1 point
- malignancy (with treatment within six months) or palliative—1.0 points

Reproduced from Wells, P.S. et al. Derivation of a simple clinical model to categorize patients' probability of pulmonary embolism: increasing the model's utility with the SimpliRED D-dimer. *Thrombosis and Haemostasis* 83(3), 416–20. DOI: 10.1055/s-0037-1613830. Copyright © 2000, Rights Managed by Georg Thieme Verlag KG Stuttgart • New York.

Depending on local guidance, the two-level Wells' score can be considered as likely (>4) or unlikely (4 or less) scores and further testing can be used to continue the risk stratification process

Further Reading

Kline JA, Mitchell AM, Kabrhel C, Richman PB, Courtney DM. Clinical criteria to prevent unnecessary diagnostic testing in emergency department patients with suspected pulmonary embolism *Journal of Thrombosis and Haemostasis*. 2004;2:1247–55.

Wells PS, Anderson DR, Rodger M, Ginsberg JS, Kearon C, Gent M, et al. Derivation of a simple clinical model to categorize patients' probability of pulmonary embolism: increasing the model's utility with the SimpliRED D-dimer. *Thrombosis and Haemostasis*. 2000;83:416–20.

SAQ 7 **Arterial Injury**

A 23-year-old female has deliberately slashed her left wrist repeatedly with a knife. It has been reported that there was active spurting of the blood at the time, which has been controlled with a pressure dressing applied by the ambulance personnel. You consider an injury to the radial artery.

Q1. List four hard signs of peripheral arterial injury.
Q2. How would you confirm the diagnosis?
Q3. What are possible complications of an unrecognized arterial injury in the limbs (list three)?

Answers

A1.

Hard signs of arterial injury include:

- Active pulsatile external haemorrhage
- Expanding or pulsatile haematoma
- Absent or reduced peripheral pulses. The presence of peripheral pulses, however, does not rule out arterial injury
- Signs of distal ischaemia (the six Ps)
- Palpable bruit or audible thrill

A2.

The diagnosis can be confirmed using a hand-held Doppler showing absence of audible arterial signals, or by ultrasonic duplex scanning. Digital pulse oximetry may help with assessment of digital perfusion. Formal wound exploration by a surgeon with vascular expertise may eventually be necessary.

A3.

An unrecognized arterial injury may lead to:

- False aneurysm formation
- Arteriovenous fistula
- Compartment syndrome

Further Reading

Fox N, Rajani RR, Bokhari F, Chiu WC, Kerwin A, Seamon MJ, et al. Evaluation and management of penetrating lower extremity arterial trauma: an Eastern Association for the Surgery of Trauma management guideline *Journal of Trauma*. 2012;73:S315–20.

SAQ 8 **Acute Calf Pain**

A 53-year-old female, with a two-day history of pain in the right calf, is referred by her general practitioner to the emergency department. The letter says, 'Please exclude deep vein thrombosis'. You note that she does not have any risk factors for venous thromboembolism and wonder if there may be an alternative explanation for her symptoms.

Q1. List three causes of acute calf pain.
Q2. On ultrasound examination, what features indicate deep vein thrombosis? List two.
Q3. What is the potential risk of anticoagulation for a person who does not have deep vein thrombosis?

Answers

A1.

Alternative causes of acute calf pain include:

- Ruptured popliteal cyst: a popliteal or Baker's cyst represents an enlargement of the gastrocnemius-semimembranosus bursa, which communicates with the knee joint
- Calf muscle strain or tear (typically involving the medial head of the gastrocnemius); this is a musculotendinous injury typically seen in middle-aged athletes participating in racquet sports (hence the name 'tennis leg'), running, and Alpine skiing
- Thrombosed popliteal aneurysm
- Cellulitis
- Superficial thrombophlebitis

A2.

In this situation, it is usual to perform a limited ultrasound examination of the common femoral vein in the groin, the proximal deep and superficial femoral veins in the thigh, and the popliteal vein in the popliteal fossa. Features of deep vein thrombosis include:

- Non-compressibility of the vein
- A persistent filling defect in the lumen caused by thrombus
- Increased diameter of the vein
- Absent colour flow
- Lack of flow augmentation on calf squeeze

A3.

There is a risk of precipitating a calf compartment syndrome if anticoagulation is inadvertently initiated, pending definitive ultrasound scanning, in a patient with a calf muscle tear or a ruptured popliteal cyst.

Further Reading

Banerjee A. The assessment of acute calf pain. *Postgraduate Medical Journal*. 1997;73:86–8.
Chung KL, Cheung KY, Kam CW. Differential diagnosis of acute calf pain and swelling with emergency ultrasound. *Hong Kong Journal of Emergency Medicine*. 2005;12:36–41.

Index

Tables, and figures, are indicated by *t*, and *f*, following the page number.

For the benefit of digital users, indexed terms that span two pages (e.g., 52–53) may, on occasion, appear on only one of those pages.